A Break in Your Cycle

A Break in Your Cycle: The Medical and Emotional
Causes and Effects of Amenorrhea © 1998 by Theresa
Francis-Cheung, MA

Library of Congress Cataloging-in-Publication Data
Francis-Cheung, Theresa
A break in your cycle / by Theresa Francis-Cheung

        p.   cm.

Includes index.

ISBN 978-1-62045-697-2

Acquiring Editor: Cheryl Kimball
Copy Editor: Renée M. Nicholls
Art/Production Manager: Claire Lewis
Text Design & Production: David Enyeart
Cover Design & Illustration: Pat Rouse

Published by
Chronimed Publishing
P.O. Box 59032
Minneapolis, MN 55459-0032

10   9   8   7   6   5   4   3   2   1

A Break in Your Cycle

A Break in Your Cycle

The Medical and Emotional Causes and Effects of Amenorrhea

Theresa Francis-Cheung, MA

CHRONIMED PUBLISHING

THERESA FRANCIS-CHEUNG, BA King's College, Cambridge University, and MA King's College, London University, is no stranger to the world of women's health. She trained and performed as a professional dancer, became a fitness teacher and consultant, taught in schools and colleges, and has also worked in health publishing.

A sufferer from menstrual dysfunction herself, she has been treated by doctors both in the United Kingdom and the United States. Currently a freelance writer, she lives in Texas with her husband, Ray.

contents

The time limit for use of the health club treadmill is thirty minutes. Mary has been running for eighty minutes now.

Lisa wears baggy clothes to conceal her body. She feels fat even though her bones are sticking out.

It is nine in the evening and Rachel is still working at the office. She arrived that morning at seven.

Linda really wants to have a baby, but she is still not pregnant a year after she stopped taking the pill.

Ninety pounds is the weight Caroline wants to drop to before she auditions for the ballet company.

Martha feels that she'll never get over the death of her parents last year.

Constantly craving food and constantly dieting, Sarah can't remember what real hunger is like anymore.

Samantha is confused and uncertain. She questions the very meaning of her life. The antidepressants that have been prescribed don't seem to be helping.

THESE WOMEN HAVE VERY DIFFERENT PROBLEMS, BUT there is one thing they all have in common. They are all suffering from amenorrhea.

Amenorrhea is the medical term for the absence or suppression of menstruation in a woman in her reproductive years who is not pregnant. Statistics reveal that the condition is on the increase as women lead increasingly stressful, complicated, and regulated lives. It is highly likely that in the twenty-first century more and more women will experience some form of amenorrhea in varying degrees of severity, from the mild (periods are absent for a few months), to the serious (periods disappear for several years or cease altogether).

Now think about your periods. Are they regular? Have you been skipping periods?

When I trained to be a dancer, when I went to study at Cambridge University, when I became a full-time fitness and exercise instructor, when I grieved for the death of my mother, and when I finally stopped taking the pill, I did not have periods. By the age of thirty, I had probably only had about twenty menstrual periods in my adult life. Because many of the professions I worked in have a high incidence of menstrual dysfunction, and I never felt unwell, it never really bothered me. But then in my early thirties I began to feel constantly despondent, weary, and irritable. To others it was obvious that my frantic lifestyle, low body weight, and terrible eating habits were probably to blame, but I was convinced that this was not the case. Being slim, working hard, proving myself, and barely resting was how I lived my life. Eventually the fatigue began to affect my work, so I reluctantly decided to make a rare visit to the doctor. One of the first questions the doctor asked was, "When did you have your last period?" It was when I told the doctor about my meager menstrual history that I first heard the word *amenorrhea.*

If you are amenorrheaic, it's likely that you also took a long time to seek out medical advice. This is easy to understand. Menstruation is still a taboo subject in our culture. It's something we all know exists, but it's also something we would rather not talk about. Even before our periods started, we were probably anxious about menstruation—convinced that it was unpleasant, that it hurt and that it was embarrassing and uncomfortable. Many of our mothers called it "the curse." So not having periods must be a blessing, right?

Menstruation as a female affliction, or a symbol of sin and evil, is the legacy that we have inherited today. The ancient idea that menstruation is a curse or a punishment for Eve's dalliance with the serpent in the garden of Eden is embedded in our history and culture.

The blood women shed every month was for centuries thought to be a sign of women's weakness and inherently demonic in nature. In some religions, a menstruating woman was considered to be unclean and to be avoided at all costs during her flow. Such beliefs continued as late as the early seventeenth century, when medical authorities still promoted the idea that menstrual blood had dark, degenerate powers.

Although much has been done, and is still being done, to change deep-seated prejudices about menstruation, the stigma still lingers.

Yet our history shows that the female reproductive cycle was not always denied or suppressed. A study of the first methods of marking time illustrates this. The earliest calendars were lunar calendars, based on the twenty-eight day cycle of the moon and the thirteen moons in the year. Since menstrual cycles follow lunar cycles, and still do today when women live away from artificial light, the strong connection between the two was emphasized. A careful study of the fragmented pieces of information that have been gathered from cultures around the world reveals that the most intimate female experiences—ovulation, menstruation, gestation, and birth—and the documenting and measuring of these events formed our ancestors' concept of time. The way a people measure time determines the timing and nature of important social functions and activities and becomes the foundation for civilization. For that reason some scholars believe that women, and not men, were the significant force behind the foundation of culture and civilization in prehistoric times.

The consequent denial of the significance and power of the menstrual cycle has created an imbalance and a distortion in our culture that is still in the process of being corrected. By contrast, in some indigenous cultures, like those of the Native American Indian, a menstruating woman is believed to have an expanded connection with universal energy at the time of her flow. This link is thought to be so powerful that it can enable a woman to bring healing to herself and the community she lives in. In other cultures, however, we have lost the basic reverence for and connection to the feminine life cycle that we once had all those centuries ago. Now we tolerate and endure menstruation rather than celebrate it for the miracle of life that it is.

Today, if we miss our periods for a while, we think, "Why complain?" No more bloating, cramping, foggy thinking! Why suffer every month if we don't have to? If we don't want to have a baby right now, what possible motivation could we have for seeing a doctor?

A Break in Your Cycle will show that although amenorrhea is not life threatening in the short term for women with normal reproductive function, it can have very serious health consequences if left untreated. If you are amenorrheaic, there is cause for concern. Until now there has been little information available that is exclusively devoted to the subject and is in terms the lay person can understand.

General books on women's health and on the menstrual cycle do sometimes have short sections on amenorrhea, but the condition, because it is so complex and has so many causes—physical, psychological, and emotional—deserves far greater attention than it has previously been given.

This study will outline what amenorrhea is, what the likely causes are, and the treatments and procedures that are available from both conventional and alternative medicine. Alongside the medical causes and effects, attention will also be paid to the emotional causes and effects, because menstruation is so much more to a woman than a simple bodily function. When a teenager starts to menstruate she begins her unique journey of self-discovery from girl to woman. How she understands and deals with her menstrual cycle at various stages in her life will indicate how she feels about herself as a woman.

Amenorrhea is a sign from your body that something is wrong. Something is out of balance. *A Break in Your Cycle* will show that, in the great majority of cases, you can combat the problem yourself and in the process gain greater health in body and mind. The key to good health often lies in the hands of the amenorrheaic herself. This book is dedicated to all women who are amenorrheaic, and also to all those who want to understand more about a condition that is of particular significance for women's issues and concerns.

acknowledgments

MY THANKS TO ALL THE MANY PEOPLE WHO HELPED provide information about amenorrhea and menstrual dysfunction in this book. In particular I would like to thank James Douglas, MD, Reproductive Endocrinologist and Infertility Specialist at the Plano Medical Center in Texas for permission to quote him and for his invaluable advice, comments, and help with research while I was writing the book. I would also like to thank all the women I have talked to over the years about amenorrhea for the insight they gave me into this complex condition. Their stories are in this book, with names and places changed to preserve identity. They provided much of the incentive to write about a condition that often goes undetected and has for too long been dismissed and ignored. I am indebted to Rachel Loos, the editor of *Company*, a women's magazine published in the United Kingdom, for her interest in this subject at a crucial time, and I am especially thankful to Cheryl Kimball, my editor at Chronimed Publishing, for her help, advice, encouragement, and insight throughout the writing process.

Thanks also to my brother, Terry, for his help with Internet research. I am also grateful for the support of friends and family. Finally, special gratitude goes to my husband, Ray, for his patience, support, enthusiasm, and love while I completed this project.

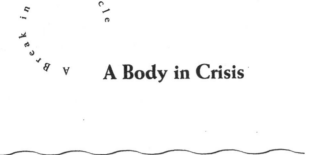

chapter 1

A Body in Crisis

~~~

ALTHOUGH AMENORRHEA IS NOT GENERALLY REGARDED as a serious medical condition, it does indicate a body in a state of crisis. So what is amenorrhea? Amenorrhea is the term used by doctors to describe the absence of the monthly flow of blood and discharge of mucous tissues from the uterus through the vagina called menstruation. Amenorrhea (*a* means without, and *menorrhea* means menstrual flow) is normal in the following cases: before sexual maturity, during pregnancy, after menstruation, in other phases of the menstrual cycle, and after menopause. It isn't normal for you to be amenorrheaic if you are between the ages of sixteen and approximately forty-five and don't fit into one of those categories. An exception to this rule would be if you have some serious defect in your reproductive system.

Amenorrhea has probably been in existence since women first walked the earth, but, along with other overlooked areas of women's health, it has been surrounded by conflict, ignorance, and confusion. Observations about failure to menstruate are not uncommon in medical history. For instance, Aetius of Amida, a sixth-century Christian physician, noticed that dancers, emaciated women, pregnant women, and singers did not menstruate. In the seventeenth century, Richard Morton's 1689 "Treatise of Consumptions" describes Mr. Duke's eighteen-year-old daughter in St. Mary Axe who became ill in July 1684:

> In the month of July she fell into a total suppression of her Monthly Courses from a multitude of Cares and Passions of her Mind.... From which time her Appetite began to abate,

and her Digestion to be bad; her Flesh also began to be flaccid and loose, and her Looks pale.

Medical practitioners in centuries past were dimly aware of the complexities of the problem, but their approach was dogmatic and often ignorant. The treatments employed, which included leeches to the vulva, scarcely bear thinking about. Mercifully we have progressed from those days, and there is far greater information available than ever before on women's health issues, but despite incredible advances, amenorrhea is still somewhat underresearched and shrouded in mystery. Why? Because it is such a complex condition. It is related not only to detectable physical disorders, such as ovarian cysts or premature ovarian failure, but also to psychological problems like stress, anxiety, and depression, which are more difficult to define. For every woman who is amenorrheaic there will be a unique cause and a unique course of treatment, and no one cure to fit all.

Types of Amenhorrhea
There are two types of amenorrhea. Primary amenorrhea is when a young woman has not started to menstruate by the age of sixteen. It is often due to low body fat, a hormonal imbalance, or a developmental problem. The last two cases can usually be treated with hormones or surgery.

Secondary amenorrhea is defined as an absence of menstruation for at least three months since the previous cycle, or sometimes as long as six months. Secondary amenorrhea more commonly affects women who have previously had normal periods. It is a very complex problem with a variety of possible causes. There is no quick answer, and it often takes a lot of time for an advisor to diagnose and treat it successfully.

A Woman's Natural Rhythm
Christiane Northrup, in her controversial but perceptive study *Women's Bodies, Women's Wisdom* (1995), emphasizes that the menstrual cycle is "the most basic earthly cycle we have." According to Northrup, the monthly bleed is our link to the "archetypal feminine." The menstrual cycle represents on a miniature scale the great macrocosmic cycles of nature, human life itself, and the universal process of change and renewal. This is why in some cultures the

menstrual cycle is revered and thought to be sacred.

Northrup believes that if you're a premenopausal woman who has menstrual dysfunction, you are in danger of losing this connection with your natural feminine rhythm, which in turn mirrors the rhythm of nature and the universe. Northrup proposes that the menstrual cycle governs not only fluids and bleeding but also the flow of knowledge, originality, and creativity in your life.

Northrup makes a valid point. There is a wisdom in the menstrual cycle. The physical changes that occur in your reproductive organs find their complement in subtle mental and emotional changes. The following brief explanation of the phases of a menstrual cycle that averages twenty-eight days will illustrate this. Please note that a woman's menstrual cycle does not always follow the typical twenty-eight-day cycle and can be much longer or shorter.)

The Menstrual Cycle

Women are born with their eggs (or ova), which are the largest cells in the body but still no bigger than a small dot. We start out with several million ova, but only a few hundred of these will mature during our life span. The ova are stored in the ovaries, oblong glands about one-and-a-half inches long. One ovary is located on each side of the pelvis.

When a girl reaches puberty, approximately every twenty-eight days an ovum will start to develop. This is called the menstrual cycle. The egg can come from either side of the body. The ovaries do not take turns maturing eggs. If one ovary is damaged or missing, the other will take over the entire workload.

The hypothalamus in the brain, the pituitary in the brain, and the ovaries are the three major glands involved in the menstrual cycle. These glands produce hormones, which are really the chemical messengers of the brain and which orchestrate the whole reproductive cycle. The release and regulation of these hormones is termed hypothalamic-pituitary-ovarian axis, or HPO axis for short. The complicated series of interrelationships that coordinate the menstrual cycle is a sophisticated chain of command that must be perfectly synchronized and coordinated for the system to run smoothly and regulate the monthly cycle. If the balance is upset in any way, menstrual dysfunction will occur.

The Follicular Phase

At the beginning of the cycle and again at day twelve, the hypothalamus produces gonadotrophin releasing hormone (GnRH), which stimulates the pituitary gland to produce follicle stimulating hormone (FSH), which in turn causes about twenty eggs in the ovaries to grow and produce the hormone estrogen. Each egg is surrounded by a sac called a follicle, and so this maturing phase is called the follicular phase. Estrogen begins to build up the lining of the uterus (or endometrium).

Studies have shown that during the follicular stage, many women report that they feel at their most bright and energetic. A new egg is growing and developing, and in our own lives we can reflect this as a time of enthusiasm, energy, ideas, and creativity.

Ovulation

The changes that occur within the ovary take place as a result of signals from the pituitary gland. The pituitary controls hormonal production in the body. It secretes its own hormones directly into the bloodstream for specialized use in the various systems of the body.

Many of the pituitary's functions are still a mystery, but it is known to operate with signals from the brain and from the rest of the body. It sends messages to the individual glands, such as the ovaries, alerting each to the needs of the systems to which the gland is associated, such as the need to produce estrogen or progesterone.

Around day ten to day fourteen of a regular twenty-eight day cycle, the pituitary produces high levels of luteinizing hormone (LH), which makes the ovaries produce more estrogen and cause ovulation. This is when one of the eggs reaches maturity, bursts out of its follicle and its ovary, is caught by the waving fingers (or fimbriae) of a fallopian tube, and starts on its journey to the uterus, or womb. By the time of ovulation this dominant follicle will have reached a size of approximately 18 to 24 millimeters. The other maturing eggs will die.

This acute rise in FSH and LH occurs at mid-cycle, usually around day fourteen of a regular twenty-eight-day cycle. Women in tune with their monthly cycle often experience ovulation as a peak of energy, sexuality, and creativity. This could perhaps be due to the hormonal surge.

A Break in Your Cycle

The Luteal Phase

The empty follicle left behind in the ovary now starts to produce another hormone called progesterone. The major function of progesterone (from the Greek word meaning *to favor birth*) is to prepare the endometrium (lining of the uterus) for implantation of a fertilized egg and for maintenance of the pregnancy. It derives from the corpus luteum, the yellow body that develops from the follicle that the mature egg was released from at ovulation. This is why the second half of the cycle is called the luteal phase. Progesterone stimulates the growth of the uterine glands, affecting the softness of the lining, and it prepares the uterine wall for implantation and support of the fertilized egg. It also maintains the life support systems of the uterus for pregnancy itself. Progesterone levels are highest around day twenty-one of a typical twenty-eight-day cycle. If fertilization does not take place, progesterone production lessens and the corpus luteum diminishes in size. As the level of progesterone wanes at the end of the cycle the uterine lining loses its support system, breaks down, and is shed in menstruation.

The luteal phase from ovulation to menstruation may make women look inward and feel more reflective. We want to retreat a little from outward activity as our bodies prepare for pregnancy (or menstruation if pregnancy does not occur). Society is not so welcoming to us in this phase, preferring us during the more outgoing, energetic, follicular phase. The premenstrual stage, often accompanied by tears, a need to be alone, and uncomfortable physical symptoms such as water retention and cramping, is the hardest phase for us to deal with. This and the sometimes painful bleeding a week or so later can seem like a curse or an illness.

There is no denying that periods can be unpleasant. At times we feel raw and sensitive. If we are not patient with ourselves during the uncomfortable times and ignore or deny our needs, we are likely to become irritable, resentful, impatient, and stressed out. However, if we manage to focus more on our inner lives during this phase in our cycle, we will discover great insight and contentment while energy stores replenish to support the next cycle of energy and creativity.

After Menstruation

Immediately after or during menstruation, FSH production increases again, stimulating follicle growth and the production of estrogen. The whole cycle begins again. Estrogen (from the Greek words *to produce desire or madness*) is commonly regarded as the female sex hormone. It influences the thickness of the uterine lining and is responsible for many female characteristics. Breast growth and development, external female genitalia, vaginal linings and secretions, and deposit of body fat are all dependent on estrogen. The hormone also has a wider effect on the whole body, influencing blood proteins, fats, and the vascular and skeletal systems. Levels of estrogen rise and fall at the command of the pituitary gland, and the fluctuations usually follow a regular pattern that coincides with stages of the menstrual cycle.

When the Balance Is Upset

Regular menstrual bleeding depends on a regular rise and fall in the hormones from the ovary and a delicate interaction between the brain and the reproductive organs at exactly the right time. It is an amazing piece of choreography, with complex moves that must be perfectly coordinated and balanced every month. If, however, for some reason the intricate balance is upset in any way, and the ovaries do not receive the right message at the right time, amenorrhea is likely to occur and menstruation will be delayed until the balance is restored.

If you are amenorrheaic, you experience none of the physical changes of a normal menstrual cycle, and therefore you experience none of the cycles of creativity, receptivity, and renewal followed by rest, reflection, and self-healing that accompany them. Every time you miss a period you lose touch with the natural feminine ebb and flow in your life and your own unique creativity.

To some extent you are existing in limbo. Not only have you broken the vital life-affirming link with your basic feminine nature, but, as later chapters will show, you are also putting your mental, physical, and emotional health at risk.

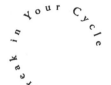

chapter 2

Women with Amenorrhea

Common Experiences

You are missing periods. You find it rather embarrassing to talk about. You think you must be the only one with this strange condition. You wonder if there might be other women out there like you.

There most certainly are! Missing a menstrual period is a lot more common than most people realize. Experiences of amenorrhea range from the mild (missing the occasional period), to the more serious (periods are absent for many months or even years). Here are some typical comments from women with amenorrhea:

> I didn't have periods when I was on the athletics team. I wasn't really worried at the time because all the women competing were the same. It was a kind of peer thing.

> I had it for six years. Nothing really worked until I saw a Chinese doctor and took these herbs. They tasted foul but they worked.

> I've just come off the pill and haven't had a period. The doctor has told me this is quite normal but I can't help but worry.

> This is a little embarrassing to confess but I didn't start my periods until I was twenty-five. I guess I must have been a very late bloomer.

> I felt a bit silly really when I went to the doctor about it. I mean most of us complain about having periods. I had to tell him that I hadn't had a period for two years. He said that I needed

to see a specialist. I haven't gotten around to making an appointment. I hate gynecologists.

I remember when I first went to college my periods stopped for months on end.

When I put on a lot of weight last year my periods seemed to disappear.

When I was a dancer ten years ago I only used to menstruate when I was on vacation.

If my weight drops below one hundred and five pounds my periods stop.

Sometimes my period is really late or I skip a month or two between periods. It's never really worried me.

Five years ago I got a fantastic promotion at work. I was terrified that I might not live up to expectations. I worked incredibly hard and skipped periods for nearly a year.

During my final years at college I was afraid that I'd fail and disappoint my whole family. During the exam terms I didn't have any periods.

In the eighties I really got into the aerobics craze. In my lunch hours and after work I would do two, maybe three, classes. I loved it—the music, the energy; but looking back my periods did become very infrequent.

When my boyfriend and I decided to go traveling after college, it was really weird. My periods stopped for months and only came back when the trip was over.

Doctors have given me pills and things but they make me feel dreadful. I wish I knew of some way to treat the problem without the pills.

The following extract, written by an amenorrhea suffer, will be published by *Company*, a leading women's magazine in the United Kingdom, along with a brief fact sheet. The fact that the editors believe it is worthy of publication, shows that the condition is far more common than many of us might think:

"I am normally a person with abundant energy and enthusiasm for life. But last year when I decided to stop taking the pill, something changed. I felt as if I was falling apart. I became distracted and unfocused; it was difficult to concentrate. I was depressed one moment, agitated the next, perpetually tired. Some days even walking up stairs was exhausting. I assured worried friends and work colleagues that my lackluster appearance was simply due to overwork. I told them all I needed was a rest and a holiday in the sun.

"Eight months later and after two holidays in the sun, all was still not well. Now even socializing with friends was becoming difficult. Most evenings all I wanted to do was to sit quietly, eat, and go to bed. This was not like me at all. In my more anxious moments I feared that I had some life-threatening disease that was slowly draining me. It really was time now to stop being stubborn and see a doctor.

"My doctor examined me and assured me I was not dying. He then asked me when I had had my last period. I told him that I had not had one since my last withdrawal bleed from the pill nearly a year ago. He then asked me a series of questions about my lifestyle, health, and diet. This was tough and I hung my head in shame. I prided myself on being an intelligent women but now I would have to confess to a diet of such obvious and grotesque malnourishment it was small wonder I was near to collapse.

"Diet Coke, coffee, chocolate, and potato chips had been the staple diet in my teens and early twenties, when I worked as a dancer. Throughout my dance career I had not menstruated but had never been concerned because this was the norm. Ballet dancers rarely have periods. Menstruation would indicate too much body fat and dancers must be light, lean, and ethereal. I aspired to this impossible ideal and the combination of vigorous exercise with insufficient food intake kept my periods absent and my weight at around a hundred pounds for a height of 5 foot 6 inches.

"When I was twenty-five I left the dance world. My body fat returned and I had normal menstrual function for two years before regulating it by going on the pill. During that time I worked as a full-time fitness instructor, averaging five to six hours of exercise a day. People used to admire my tremendous energy and slim physique. I wonder now if I was paying the price for those exciting but frenzied years.

"The doctor to my relief did not reprimand me. He simply informed me that I had secondary amenorrhea. I had never heard of the word and discovered that it is the medical term used to describe the absence of normal menstrual function.

"Whatever relief I had about not being on my deathbed was quickly eclipsed by my understanding of amenorrhea. I did not know whether to laugh or cry. Wasn't the absence of menstruation some kind of precursor to menopause? Hold on, I wanted to shout. This can't be happening. I'm too young. I'm only thirty. Was the goddess of fertility finally exacting her revenge for all the years I had abused my body and pushed it to the limits?

"Or was my amenorrhea the consequence, not of poor diet and overexercise, but of taking the pill for four years? The doctor said that probably a combination of many factors had caused the hormonal imbalance I was suffering from. He explained that many women do experience some kind of post-pill amenorrhea before normal menstruation returns. Usually this lasts no more than a few months but in some cases it could be longer. The doctor told me not to worry, to eat a more balanced and healthy diet and to come back in six months.

"My husband assured me that everything would be all right. I appreciated his sympathy but wondered how he could ever understand what it felt like to be a woman without her natural, feminine rhythms. Having only just been married for a year I never knew what to say when friends kept asking when, or if, we were going to start a family. Amenorrhea was robbing me of the right to even choose. Without menstruation I was infertile.

"I tried to get on with my life as normal, but fears of tumors, early menopause and irreversible infertility (absent menstruation is a symptom for all these conditions) flashed through my mind. I grew more miserable daily and lost my confidence and sense of humor. Socializing became a trauma. I felt a failure as a woman…"

Common Concerns

If you are amenorrheaic, it is probable that even if you have consulted a doctor you are still bewildered and uncertain about the condition, what causes it, and how best to treat it. Your concerns might be similar to these:

A Break in Your Cycle

I usually get my period every three weeks. But it has been seven weeks now and I haven't gotten it. Pregnancy is not an option because I haven't had sexual intercourse. So what is the problem? Should I be worried?

What is the usual treatment for missed periods? I haven't had my period for half a year (since I stopped taking the pill). I have also lost some weight. What are the health effects of missed periods?

I haven't had any menstrual period for five months. I don't take drugs and I'm not pregnant. What is the problem?

I am thirty years old and I have not had any periods for the last eleven years. Last year the doctor prescribed birth control pills, which did cause me to have my period but I suffered horrible side effects (vomiting, severe mood swings). As a result I stopped taking the pills because no matter how low the hormonal dosage, I suffered the side effects. I would like to know if there is any other way to treat amenorrhea.

I'm only thirty-six and my periods have stopped. Am I in early menopause? Is there anything I can do about it?

I had anorexia in my teens and did not menstruate. I went down to seventy pounds and had to be hospitalized. I'm finally dealing with my eating disorder, but I really need to know if I have ruined my chances of ever starting a family?

I don't menstruate. Does that mean I'm infertile?

Should I stop exercising altogether to get my periods back?

I've read that women with HIV get amenorrhea. Should I get myself tested?

I'm scared. Have I got some kind of tumor?

I feel bloated a lot these days. Where is all my menstrual blood going? It can't be right that I'm not getting rid of it any more. My body must be full of toxins.

The drugs the doctors prescribed for depression make me feel better but should I tell him that they have stopped my periods?

The doctor says I should just relax, eat better, and my periods should come back. Is that really the case or is there something seriously wrong with me?

Have I got a problem with my thyroid gland or my kidneys? Is that stopping my periods?

I am the right weight for my build, so low body fat can't be causing my amenorrhea. What is then?

Should I seek help from conventional or alternative medicine for my lack of menstruation?

The questions seem endless. Doctors do try to explain, but if you are anxious about being amenorrheaic, there is simply not enough information and guidance available. You may find it hard to discuss the issue with friends and partners. You may feel excluded—cut off from women's gossip, bonding, and empathy for "that time of the month." You may not feel so sexy and feminine anymore. You know something is not right but you do not know what to do about it.

You may wonder why you are in this situation in the first place. Is it your fault? Is it a disease? Why have your ovaries shut down? Have they forgotten what to do? What a scary thought. Your body has forgotten how to be female. Your fertility is sleeping. Will your ovaries ever wake up again and do their job?

Because so little information is available on amenorrhea, it is easy to conclude that it must be a very rare condition indeed. This is definitely not the case, but sufferers often feel isolated and confused, making the situation worse. What is needed is greater awareness and understanding of amenorrhea. This is slowly beginning to happen as research leads to better treatment options from doctors and therapists, but there is still a way to go.

Additional Sources of Information

Women's magazines, which so often reflect the trends in women's concerns and interest, are finally starting to publicize amenorrhea and the problems and complications it can cause. The following are extracts taken from articles found in leading women's and fitness magazines. The full articles are brief, but the fact that they were published is a positive development and shows how awareness is growing:

It is not uncommon for competitive female athletes to have a loss of menstruation. This phenomena is called amenorrhea. (Kelting 1988)

Kelting's article discusses how when a woman's total body fat reaches a low level, her ability to produce estrogen is affected and amenorrhea occurs. It associates amenorrhea with eating disorders and malnutrition and suggests that it can cause emotional and psychological problems for women who wish to conceive.

To maintain menstruation, women need a certain amount of calories, protein and body fat. In addition, factors such as stress, weight loss, intense training, a history of irregular periods and late menarche can make a woman more prone to the cessation of menstruation. Amenorrhea is a warning from your body that there is too much energy drain. (Otis and Goldingay 1992)

Forsyth's article "Amenorrhea: What Your Body Is Trying to Tell You" suggests that the most common cause of amenorrhea is over-exercise combined with poor eating habits. It says that all underweight women are at risk, especially those with eating disorders such as anorexia. The article then stresses the danger of early onset osteoporosis, a gradual reduction in the amount of bone mass for amenorrheaic women. (Forsyth 1993)

Warning to women runners: Just because you menstruate regularly does not mean all is well in the land of fertility. Though amenorrhea is known to impair fertility, researchers have found that more subtle menstrual irregularities may have a similar effect. ("Running Away from Motherhood." 1993)

Amenorrhea strikes up to 20 percent of women who exercise vigorously and as many as one-half of all serious runners. (Cohen 1994)

Cohen's article shows that the standard explanation for amenorrhea—too much exercise produces too little body fat, reducing estrogen production and causing menstruation to cease—is not the whole story. Poor nutrition can also cause amenorrhea, and the condition appears to be related to inadequate energy supply.

Hoffman's article "Your Period: How Normal Is It?" includes

information on amenorrhea and irregular menstrual function (Hoffman 1995).

> Though many women may welcome the cessation of menstruation each month, it should never be a goal. Amenorrhea is a dangerous condition because the female body is in crisis mode. (Hogg 1997)

Hogg's insightful article shows how energy deficiency can cause amenorrhea and how frustrating the problem can be for sufferers, because there is no quick remedy. According to the author, doctors too often look at the symptoms and not at the underlying problems that cause amenorrhea. It suggests that although poor diet and overexercise are contributory factors, what really needs to be investigated is the patient's psychological state, emphasizing the mind-body link. It shows that treatments that try to understand the patient's attitudes are now available, and that they have a greater success rate than treatments that neglect or ignore the patient's state of mind.

Levine's article "Am I Normal or Is Something Seriously Wrong?" includes related information on the menstrual cycle and irregular bleeding. (Levine 1997)

Moving Forward

Amenorrhea is much more common than many of us realize. If you are amenorrheaic, you shouldn't feel you are alone. Women from all walks of life can be victims of the disorder and there is treatment and advice available.

The very fact that you are reading this book demonstrates that you are aware of the problem and want to learn more about its complexities. Gaining awareness is always the first step on the road to recovery. The following chapters will explain the causes and effects, both physical and psychological; help you assess the various treatment options available; and encourage you to help yourself by thinking about your own lifestyle and how it might, in fact, be contributing to the problem.

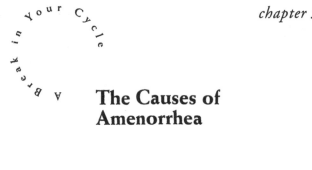

chapter 3

The Causes of Amenorrhea

AMENORRHEA IS NOT A DISEASE OF THE REPRODUCTIVE system, but it is a symptom of another disorder. In the great majority of instances, a primary disease or an imbalance is causing the secondary problem of amenorrhea. In all cases, amenorrhea has its own risks and should never be ignored.

It isn't easy for doctors to find out the primary cause of amenorrhea without extensive testing and research. The disorder is complex, and it can be caused by physical or psychological problems. This is what makes it so difficult to treat. There are almost as many causes as there are women who are amenorrheaic.

In this chapter I will first discuss the times in our lives when being amenorrheaic is perfectly natural. I will then mention some of the rare anatomical disorders that can prevent menstruation. Finally, I will explain how a disorder in the endocrine system can result in amenorrhea. An endocrine or hormonal disorder is by far the most common cause of absent periods, so I will discuss this in greater detail in the chapters that follow.

Natural Causes

There are times in our lives when amenorrhea is not an ominous sign and is perfectly natural: before puberty, during pregnancy, while breast-feeding, immediately following menstruation until the next period, and during and after menopause.

It is only in the last hundred years or so that the great majority of women have experienced monthly periods for a substantial part of their lives. There are many reasons for this. We are living longer. Menopause is reached later, and puberty is reached earlier. Lifestyle and diet changes and better standards of living encourage regular, healthy menstruation. Our malnourished ancestors had a far higher incidence of miscarriage, amenorrhea, infertility, and stillbirth than we have today. The average family size has also declined. In the days before birth control a woman could be in a constant state of amenorrhea due to pregnancy, breast-feeding, or recovery from miscarriage.

Before Puberty

Before the days of artificial lighting, the mean age of first menstruation (called *menarche*) was fourteen or fifteen. For modern girls, the mean age of menarche is now eleven or twelve, and it is getting earlier and earlier.

Earlier menarche is due, among other things, to a change in society's eating habits. The twentieth-century diet is high in fat that contains both the estrogens used to fatten animals and estrogen-mimicking chemicals. Estrogen is essential for healthy menstrual function.

Another influential factor is the use of artificial light to replace natural light. The rhythm of the menstrual cycle is organized through the interlacing of hormones that work in tandem with the pineal and pituitary glands, the brain, the ovaries, and the uterus. The pituitary is stimulated by a variety of influences, such as emotions, sex, and nutrition, and this in turn is acted upon by another gland deep within the brain called the pineal gland, which secretes the neurohormone melatonin. The pineal gland responds to changes in light/dark cycles and orchestrates the bodily rhythms. This gland will send the body a signal when the time is ripe for the secretion of hormones that bring about puberty, the transitional stage between childhood and full maturity. In centuries past, when the sun went down the only source of light available was soft candlelight. With the invention of electricity, life changed dramatically. Today, a young girl will have a greater amount of light stimulation, and this may cause her to reach puberty at a younger age. She can expect to spend at least the next thirty years of her life with a monthly menstrual bleed. Amenorrheaic women, however, break this cycle. Primary amenorrheaics postpone the onset of menstruation for many years, into their late teens or early twenties, and secondary amenorrheaics suspend menstrual function for any number of months or years.

Normally, with the onset of puberty, the nipples begin to enlarge. This is closely followed by an enlargement of the external genitalia, pubic hair, breast development, and a growth spurt. Later, vaginal secretions will indicate that menstruation is about to begin. The preparation of the ovaries for reproductive function is somehow triggered by changes in body fat, and well before menarche, hypothalamic-releasing factors begin to stimulate the secretion of FSH and LH by the pituitary gland. Estrogen production begins until there is enough for menstruation.

If you are suffering from primary amenorrhea, the most probable explanation is that you are lacking enough estrogen and other hormones to trigger the onset of puberty. You will be getting older, but like Peter Pan, you are not really growing up. If you have secondary amenorrhea and have passed puberty, absent menses could indicate that you have reverted back to abnormal or more immature hormone levels. Your body may have gone into reverse gear, returning to the prepubertal state in a hormonal holding pattern.

During Pregnancy and Breast-Feeding

One obvious reason for missing a period is that you are expecting. This is the first conclusion that doctors, friends, and family will jump to if you mention the problem, and it is one that can cause a great deal of embarrassment or disappointment. If you have been sexually active, then it is vital that pregnancy be ruled out as soon as possible as the cause, even if you have not been menstruating. Although it is unlikely, women who have been amenorrheaic for several months or years can get pregnant. Studies have shown that a woman can spontaneously ovulate at any time in her cycle, even during menstruation itself. This could be in response to any number of factors. Women have been known to ovulate, for instance, at the sight of a loved one, when their eating habits change, when there is a change in their lifestyle, and at times of extreme emotion. There is really no "safe" time to have sex, and being amenorrheaic does not mean you have an effective form of contraceptive. It is extremely important to diagnose pregnancy early so that decisions can be made for the benefit and health of both child and mother, if the pregnancy is to continue, and for an early abortion to be arranged if the pregnancy is unwanted.

Women who are pregnant do not menstruate because the fall in hormone support from the ovary to the uterus that causes menstruation does not occur. Instead, the lining remains and hormone activity continues in order to protect and support the growing fetus. During breast-feeding, a woman also remains amenorrheaic. High levels of prolactin, the hormone that prepares the breast for lactation, suppresses the menstrual function.

After Menopause

Usually, between the ages of forty and fifty a woman's ovaries start to make fewer hormones. They begin to reverse how they functioned in the early years of reproductive life during puberty. The eventual cessation of ovulation and the menstrual cycle is due to this waning level of ovarian (hormonal) output. This process can take several years, and the years leading up to the last menstrual period a woman will have are now referred to as the perimenopause.

At present, the average age of menopause is around fifty, but it ranges from the ages of forty-five to fifty-five, although some women go through it in their late thirties or even earlier. The ovaries eventually cease to function without hormonal support, and the uterine lining stops shedding every month in menstruation. Amenorrhea becomes permanent, and the transition that is menopause has occurred. For the rest of her life, a woman will not have a menstrual period, and she will no longer be able to bear children. Frequently, this stage in life is accompanied by physical symptoms as the body adjusts to the hormonal shifts taking place. These include profuse sweating, mood shifts, and changes in appetite and sleep patterns.

The key to a successful transition through menopause lies in each woman's attitude toward it. Once again, though, we are not helped by the fact that much of what is said about menopause tends to cast a negative light on the experience. Many of us still find it hard to deny that what is referred to as the "change in life" seems more like the end of life. We think of stereotypical images of bitter, vindictive, jealous, neurotic, and impossible old women suffering psychological disorders that manifest in strange symptoms such as hot flashes, depression, and irritable behavior. Unconsciously we are terrified of menopause and wonder how we will cope. We regard it not as a natural process but as part of the aging and declining process. The reproductive organs start to atrophy, so surely it will not be long before the rest of us does too.

The idea that menopause means getting old and no longer having a role to fulfill in society is obsolete due to changes in cultural attitudes and advances in medical research. In today's society, a woman's importance is no longer measured and defined solely in terms of childbearing. Important medical research has also shown that the uncomfortable feelings that accompany menopause are not due to decline or decay but to hormonal factors. The common physical discomforts of menopause, both sexual and emotional, result indirectly or directly from a lack of estrogen or progesterone. Lack of estrogen causes the typical menopausal symptoms: migraines, nausea, hot flashes, insomnia, mood swings, and loss of sex drive, which—because they tend to be vague and hard to describe—were once thought to be "all in the head."

If you can successfully negotiate your way through the remaining vestiges of negativity surrounding attitudes about menopause, you will discover that it can be a positive experience. "I consider menopause a second puberty, an initiation into what can be the most powerful, exciting, and fulfilling half of a woman's life," writes Joan Borysenko in her insightful study *A Woman's Book of Life* (1992). Free from the reproductive cycle, women at this stage in life have the opportunity to fully understand themselves, their sexuality, the source of their own power, and what they have to contribute to the world. The wise woman in all of us can finally emerge, confident, insightful, and a source of power for ourselves and others.

There are dramatic and often difficult physical, emotional, and psychological changes to encounter at menopause, but it is still, as Borysenko states, "powerful, exciting and fulfilling." We can find real fulfillment both personally and socially, and we can engage in mutually satisfying relationships that are both sexual and nonsexual. Just because a woman cannot bear children does not mean that she cannot be sexual. It is time that we separate reproductive function from sexual potential. Seen in this light, menopause is not an ending but a dynamic and challenging beginning for us all.

Anatomical Causes

A congenital defect refers to something a person is born with. Something goes wrong in the development of the baby in the womb, and the child is born with an anomaly, a variation from the norm. Sometimes women who are amenorrheaic are born with defects or without a vagina or uterus (womb). Some of these conditions are listed in this section.

Absence of the Uterus or Vagina

You will be amenorrheaic if you don't have a uterus. (If you have had any sort of menstrual bleeding in your life it is highly unlikely that this is the cause of your amenorrhea.) When the uterus and vagina are absent due to a birth defect, the ovaries may still be functioning or working normally. Puberty takes place because hormones are present and eggs begin to form but there is no menstruation because there is no uterus to bleed from. Primary amenorrhea occurs even though breasts and pubic hair are developing normally.

Disorders of Sexual Differentiation

A hermaphrodite has attributes that are both male and female. Named after the mythic Hermaphroditus from his fusion with the nymph Salmacis, the true hermaphrodite has both an ovary and a testis, sometimes on opposite sides and sometimes included in the same gland. The end result is a puzzle. The child is born with abnormal genitals that display the gender confusion. True hermaphrodites are rare. Much more common is pseudohermaphrodism, a condition in which patients have either testes or ovaries but still have ambiguous-looking genitals or some other confusion about whether they are male or female.

Hermaphrodism is a distressing and difficult area for both patients and doctors to deal with requiring time, patience, and emotional, mental, and physical adjustment to whatever sex is finally decided on. Whenever there is doubt about ascribing gender at birth, "female" tends to be the safer option: when it comes to sex, an absent vagina can be corrected by surgery whereas a penis cannot. These patients will be amenorrheaic.

Testicular Feminization

Sometimes during gestation the necessary sensitivity to the male hormone testosterone required for a normal, functioning female does not occur and the testes remain, as well as a vagina and vulva. This condition is called testicular feminization. At birth the girl looks normal. She develops breasts in puberty, but menstruation does not occur because the testes have suppressed the development of a uterus. The condition is genetic, and the child should be raised as a girl. Needless to say, she will not menstruate.

Lower Brain Adhesions
This is an extremely rare cause of amenorrhea. A very few women are born with a lower brain that does not function properly. They cannot get pregnant. These women are usually short and underdeveloped.

Turner's Syndrome
A rare genetic abnormality characterized by ovaries that contain no eggs is called Turner's Syndrome. The stigmas of Turner's Syndrome include shortness of stature, a shieldlike chest, a webbed neck, short fourth metacarpals and metatarsals, and congenital heart disease. Lacking normal ovarian hormones, these patients do not go through puberty and do not develop sexual characteristics. They are amenorrheaic and cannot have children in the normal way. The abnormality is caused by defects in the genetic blueprint.

Transverse Vaginal Septum
Some women are born with another kind of complication. The uterus is either partially or completely divided by a wall called a septum. Called a separate uterus, this causes delayed menarche and pelvic pain. Treatment is necessary to correct the problem and is often successful.

Imperforate Hymen
This transverse barrier across the lower part of the vagina can come about as an abnormality at birth, but sometimes it can occur after an inflammation in early childhood causes the bits of the normal hymen to stick together. It is often hard to detect the problem until puberty, when periods are due to begin. Amenorrhea often manifests itself as a symptom. If bleeding does occur, there is hidden amenorrhea or cryptomenorrhea. Cryptomenorrhea is apparent amenorrhea resulting from an obstruction to menstruation, such as an imperforate hymen or a transverse vaginal septum. The blood accumulates under the blockage and the vagina distends,

causing great pain every month that will only get worse. Treatment is vital and, once performed, usually successful.

Adhesions and Infections

There will be no menstrual cycle if the uterus or uterus lining has been destroyed by infection or adhesions.

Endometritis

Endometritis—destruction of the uterine cavity by infection—is not to be confused with endometriosis, a condition associated with infertility. Endometritis means inflammation of the endometrium, usually from an infection. The inflammation develops rapidly as part of another, more dominant, infection. Tuberculosis endometritis is one of the most common causes of amenorrhea in certain parts of the world, but it is not so common in the West. Treatment is possible in certain cases.

Asherman's Syndrome

Sometimes women form adhesions after a dilation of the cervix of the uterus and scraping (curettage) of the endometrium (lining) of the uterus (womb). This operation is often called a D&C. Other operations that carry a slight risk of adhesions within the uterus are those to repair a malformed uterus and those that try to remove fibroids within the uterine cavity. These adhesions are called Asherman's Syndrome, and they are caused by an overvigorous scraping of the uterus. Amenorrhea is one of the first signs of Asherman's Syndrome.

Adjusting to Irreversible Amenorrhea

A girl born with congenital absence of the uterus or vagina, or with a genetic anomaly, will need a lot of understanding and assistance. It is impossible to give her a uterus, although it is possible to fashion a vagina from the soft tissue that appears where the uterus would be. She will never be able to have a baby. But she may have normal ovaries and normal hormones, and there is no physical reason why she should not lead a healthy, active normal life and engage in sexual relationships. Adoption and surrogate motherhood are options she can consider.

On the other hand, coming to terms with the situation emotionally may take a lot of time. This will also be true in the case of women who have become irreversibly amenorrheaic due to complications or infections or who have had a hysterectomy (an operation in which the womb is surgically removed). If you have irreversible amenorrhea, it is more important than ever that you make a distinction in your mind between being sexual and feminine and having reproductive capacity. You are still a woman in every sense of the word. Creating a baby is not an option, but having a creative, fulfilling life that enriches you and others is.

Endocrine Causes

Anatomical problems that cause amenorrhea are actually quite rare. Far more common is amenorrhea caused by complications in the endocrine system, including the hypothalamus, pituitary, adrenal, and ovarian glands. After a brief description here, these will be discussed more fully in the next few chapters.

The term endocrine system refers to the group of endocrine glands that produce and secrete hormones directly into the bloodstream. The hormones then travel to specific organs and exert their influence. Figure 1 on the next page illustrates how the hypothalamic-pituitary-ovarian feedback system that regulates menstruation normally operates. Readers may also wish to review the discussion on pages 15 through 18.

The Hypothalamus

What happens in the uterus is dependent on secretions from the ovary. The ovary is stimulated in turn by secretions from the pituitary. The marvelous chain of command does not stop there. The pituitary is controlled by the hypothalamus. The hypothalamus regulates the production and secretion of pituitary hormones by producing its own hormones in nerve cells, called GnRH (gonadotropin releasing hormone). GnRH stimulates the release of follicular-stimulating releasing hormone and luteinizing hormone releasing hormone from the pituitary gland, both of which will stimulate the ovaries.

Not much bigger than a thimble, the hypothalamus in the lower brain is constantly alert and regulates bodily functions such as hunger, thirst, growth, sleep, body temperature, and reproduction. It also indirectly controls thyroid and adrenal function. The thyroid

FIGURE I

Hypothalamic-Pituitary-Ovarian Axis

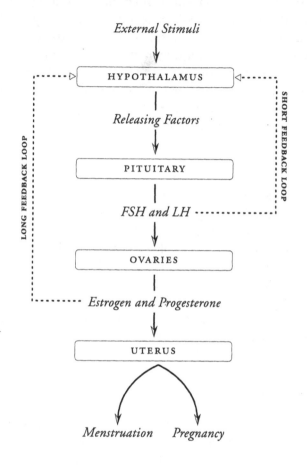

gland regulates metabolic rate, and the adrenal glands secrete hormones that help us respond to stress. Both glands can influence ovarian function.

The crucial thing to understand is that the hypothalamus is the bridge connecting the nervous system (brain) with the endocrine system (bodily secretions) and the reproductive cycle. It receives input from the higher centers in the brain, which in themselves are modified and influenced by the outside world. Any number of internal or external factors can affect the function of the hypothalamus. For instance, emotional stress, environmental factors, changes in blood hormone levels, and certain drugs may alter the hormone-secreting nerve cells of the hypothalamus and influence the menstrual cycle.

To recap, the incredible control system regulating the menstrual cycle is dependent on the interrelationships of the hypothalamus, the pituitary, the ovaries, and the uterus. But other factors, within or outside the body, can influence the intricate balance of hormones and the delicate timing of the whole system. Malfunction can occur when disease affects one of the major systems, such as a tumor in the pituitary gland. It can also occur when chronic stress disturbs the hypothalamus because the hypothalamus indirectly controls thyroid, adrenal, and pituitary functions that influence the menstrual clock. When the balance of this perfectly synchronized endocrine system is upset, the reproductive cycle becomes disturbed or shuts down altogether, and the condition known as hypothalamic amenorrhea will occur.

Hypothalamic Amenorrhea

This condition takes place when ovulation does not occur because no egg is released from the ovary every month due to a lack of hormonal stimulation by the HPO axis. The most common menstrual sequel to this failure to ovulate (or anovulation), is amenorrhea, although in some cases enough estrogen is still produced to cause irregular menstrual bleeding, a condition called oligomenorrhea.

One fairly common cause of hypothalamic anovulation or hypothalamic amenorrhea is stress. The various kinds of stresses, both physical and psychological, that can influence the menstrual clock will be examined in the next chapter.

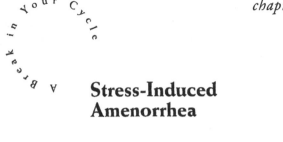

chapter 4

Stress-Induced Amenorrhea

WHEN HORMONAL IMBALANCE IS A FACTOR, THERE IS often a very thin line between a physical and a psychological cause. What caused what? Did state of mind or stress create an imbalance, or was the problem caused by a bodily disorder that then influenced state of mind and caused stress? Research has proved that how we think and feel does influence our body's chemistry. This certainly is so with amenorrhea. Studies indicate that if lifestyle changes are not made, the disorder will simply return after medical treatment has been administered to induce menstruation. It is possible to have a set of attitudes that can predispose you to problems with menstruation. When you miss periods, your body is telling you that it is in conflict with these attitudes, thoughts, and feelings, and that you need to alter the way you act, think, and feel in some way.

Hypothalamic amenorrhea is usually the result of stress. Intense emotions and stressful situations affect the brain's biochemistry, which in turn disrupts hypothalamus function. Basically, stress causes control center malfunction in the hypothalamus. The right signals are not sent out at the right time to regulate and control the menstrual cycle. No GnRH is released from the hypothalamus, the pituitary is not stimulated, and consequently no FSH and LH is released to regulate the menstrual cycle. With such an inadequate drive to the ovaries, proper development of the follicles stops and ovulation cannot occur.

Stress

There is not a human being alive who does not know something about stress. It has become a part of everyday life. Environmental factors, such as changes in climate, physical problems and illnesses, emotional upsets, job pressures, financial constraints, family difficulties, and even vacations themselves can all cause stress. Most of us are not even aware of stress because our bodies have methods of adapting. If stress is extreme, however, or if it continues for a long period of time, the body is not so good at counterbalancing. It is then that stress can cause harm to your body. When the hypothalamus is bombarded with stress, even though your reproductive system is normal, ovulation will stop and menses will cease.

The first reaction of our body to extreme danger or threat of bodily harm is called the flight or fight response. This very human reaction dates back to a time when life was a constant struggle for survival. Think about how you react when you are frightened or upset or threatened. You are no different from your ancient ancestors. Like them, your heart will pound, your blood pressure will rise, your muscles will tense, and your eyes will open wide. This cluster of reactions alerts all your body systems to the apparent danger and helps you make the next step, which is either to resist or fight.

Of course, not all stressful events are so sudden or so obvious as the threat of bodily harm. Any challenge that overwhelms us—a serious illness, the death of a loved one, the loss of a job, the end of a relationship—can be stressful enough to cause hypothalamic dysfunction.

The following list, developed from "The Social Readjustment Scale" by Holmes and Rale (1967) is often used by doctors to rate situations that are most likely to cause stress for both men and women. These situations are rated from most stress to least stress.

- Death of a spouse
- Divorce
- Marital separation
- Jail term
- Death of a close family member
- Personal injury or illness
- Marriage
- Fired at work

- Marital reconciliation
- Retirement
- Change in health of a family member
- Pregnancy
- Sexual difficulties
- Gain of a new family member
- Business adjustment
- Change in financial state
- Death of a close friend
- Change to a different line of work
- Change in number of arguments with spouse
- Large mortgage
- Foreclosure of mortgage or loan
- Change in responsibilities at work
- Son or daughter leaving home
- Trouble with in-laws
- Outstanding personal achievement
- Wife begins or stops work
- Begin or end school or college
- Change in living conditions
- Revision of personal habits
- Trouble with boss
- Change in work hours or conditions
- Change in residence
- Change in schools
- Change in recreation
- Change in church activities
- Change in social activities
- Small mortgage
- Change in sleeping habits
- Change in number of family get-togethers
- Change in eating habits
- Vacation
- Christmas
- Minor violations of the law

Certain events, like death or divorce, are obviously traumatic, but the list demonstrates that there are many other events and situations that are less obviously stressful. A change in routine of any sort, for instance in eating habits or in travel arrangements, will challenge the body as it tries to adapt to the new way of doing things, and sometimes even activities thought pleasurable, like weddings or Christmas, can be stressful.

We all have different ways of coping with the stresses in our lives. It is not the events in themselves, as difficult as some of them may be, that cause the problem, but how we cope with and respond to them. Some of us are more vulnerable to stressful situations or events, while others are more productive in how they respond to stress. In the words of Joan Borysenko, in *Minding the Body, Mending the Mind* (1987) it depends on our constitutions: "Most of us will feel that life is out of control in some way. Whether we see this as a temporary situation whose resolution will add to our store of knowledge and experience or as one more threat demonstrating life's dangers is the most crucial question both for the quality of our life and our physical health." Those of us with a more heightened sensitivity to stress, with a more tense, anxious, and worrying nature than others, are more likely to suffer from amenorrhea.

Stress occurs when there is an imbalance between the demands of your life and your ability to cope with it. Continued stress over a long period of time will deplete the body's resources, producing fatigue, changes in appetite, insomnia, depression, and amenorrhea. If your periods have stopped, it could be a sign that stress levels are too high in your life. Unrelieved stress is very dangerous. It can diminish the body's immune system, making you more vulnerable to disease. It may also bring on hypertension, a recognized factor in heart disease and some cancers.

The way to avoid stress altogether would be to do nothing at all, but this is no way to live. All our actions, thoughts, and feelings involve some kind of stress. Some stresses, though, like planning a wedding or playing a game of tennis, are fulfilling and stimulating. Stress is not necessarily always bad for you—quite the reverse. Provided you are fit and healthy enough to cope with it, a positive kind of stress, at a level that does not make you feel uncomfortable, is the vital ingredient your life needs to be make it energetic and exciting. It is negative stress, stress that is excessive and draining, that results in anxiety and eventual mental and physical breakdown. This is the kind of stress to avoid. Some examples of the kinds of situations that can cause negative stress, impact hypothalamic function, and make your periods stop are discussed in this section.

Stressful Professions

Mandy sighed. Nobody was really watching her as she signaled which way the exits were. If only they'd pay more attention, she thought. They have no idea how important these instructions are. As she motioned from left to right, it all came back to her. The yelling, the shouting, the blood, the panic, the fear. That was five years ago. She said she would never work on planes again but here she was on Flight 216A to France.

It was a busy cabin, and Mandy knew that with the chronic staff shortage she would barely get a chance to sit down for the next six hours at least. She fastened her seat belt as the plane took off, and yawned, trying to get her ears to pop. She hadn't quite recovered from her trip to Australia yet. It surprised her that after all these years she still hadn't gotten used to hours and days disappearing, merging into one as time zones were crossed. She took a deep breath and looked at the passengers: lots of children, and several VIPs to pamper in rows 10A and 10B. Her nose felt a little runny. She was sure she was getting a cold, but there was no time to think about that now. She had a job to do and the passengers needed to see a smiling face.

Working in certain professions, like being a firefighter, a doctor, or an operator of dangerous machinery, can be stressful if our mental and physical constitutions are not strong enough to deal with them. Flight attendants, like Mandy, frequently have irregular or absent periods. It's a stressful job, dealing with a demanding public, and the hypothalamus is constantly bombarded by noise pollution, high altitudes, and changes in light cycle. Long flights across time zones where the sun rises at different hours affect the hypothalamus and consequently have an impact on ovulation.

Overwork

Sarah, age thirty-two, has a remarkable career. A Harvard University graduate in law, she fell into journalism as a behind-the-scenes expert and has worked in New York and Washington for ten years. The assignments she is given are all-consuming; she has no time for anything else. She rarely takes a day off and is under constant pressure to reach deadlines. She often feels drained, exhausted, and frustrated by the internal political dynamics of her profession. She knows she needs to take a vacation, but last year she cut short her vacation, fearing that she might miss out on something important at work. Sarah has been amenorrheaic for three years.... She hasn't sought treatment, although she keeps intending to because the condition does worry her.

Job Insecurity

"Even if I rise to the top of my profession," says Sally, age thirty-two, and a finance executive, "even if I am tough, even if I do my job, by the slight flick of a finger my boss could still fire me, or stop me from progressing any further within the company by rating my performance badly. There's always the insecurity in my job. What would happen if one day I did bungle things. I dread losing a big customer. I'm scared that so many things might appear on my record, stand against me. I'm always scared I'll make a big mistake. I have to be so careful when I go to the corporate parties. My husband has to behave properly, 'cause we have to fit in the mold. You've got to be on guard." Sally has been amenorrheaic for ten months.

Amenorrhea is the body's response to constant fear and worry. Financial hardship, unemployment, and the threat of unemployment can cause emotional and physical stress.

Relationships

Louise cried for six months when he left her. Sometimes she missed him so much it hurt, but at other times she felt that she was in control, especially now that her periods had stopped. She didn't need to think about Roger anymore. She was strong. She didn't need anyone. Nobody was ever again going to hurt her like he did.

Rebecca, eighteen, sat alone crying. She wasn't eating anymore, she wasn't menstruating anymore, and she didn't care. She had lost the most important person in her life, her sister. Never a day went by when she wouldn't reach to pick up the phone for their daily chats and have to stop herself. It had all been so sudden: the car crash, then the funeral. She had been strong for everyone else, but now terrible nightmares of the crash tortured her. At times she felt so inconsolable and lonely she wished there was something she could take to make the pain go away.

Our relationships with other people are also a source of stress. Problems with our partners, our family, our friends, and our colleagues can cause anxiety. Relationships are life sustaining but they can also make us very vulnerable. Divorce or the death of a loved one sometimes shocks the system as much as a physical blow.

Change of Residence

Helen moved from London to New York with her husband. She really thought the move would be an easy transition—at least there was not a new language to learn. She soon realized how wrong she was. Everything about the American way of life was different and it took a long time to adjust. She felt isolated and misunderstood and for nine months her periods stopped.

Adapting to a new way of life is never easy. Moving is high on the list of stress-inducing circumstances. In a very short space of time you have to get used to a whole new way of life. Everything that was known is replaced by a whole new set of rules and people. You feel vulnerable and nervous as you try to establish yourself, unsure of where to go, what to do, what to say. You miss the old way of life. Your body is trying to adapt to the new routine, and in the process menstrual health may suffer.

Travel

There was no doubt Chloe's trip to India had been an incredible experience. She had the most fantastic memories. It hadn't been without its stresses, though. Like the constant diarrhea and the bouts of illness. She had survived the trip, but her periods hadn't. She'd been back for three months now and still no period.

Travel can also unsettle the status quo and cause complications.

Seasonal Variation

Mary used to enjoy her morning runs, but when her shift changed at work she had to run in the evenings instead. As winter drew close she found more often than not that she would have to run in the dark. Her periods became irregular and didn't stabilize again until spring.

Ovarian function can be affected by seasonal variation. Decreased ovarian activity in autumn can sometimes be related to an increased pineal secretion of melatonin. The conception rate of women living in Northern Scandinavia is actually higher during the summer than in the winter. Runners who run in the dark, or in autumn and winter, have an increased incidence of amenorrhea. Daylight and sunshine seem to favor ovulation.

Hard Living

"The conditions in Auschwitz were indescribably wretched. The prisoners were given hardly anything to eat and no medicines were available. Hundreds died from starvation and illness every day. The guards beat and clubbed people to death for no reason at all. Every day new groups of prisoners were sent to the gas chambers. No one could be sure of his or her life. Every day could be the last...." (Van der Rol and Verhoeven, 1995)

In times of war, famine, and crisis menstrual function is impacted. It is a well-documented fact that the women who endured the Nazi war camps, and the terrible degradation and cruelty inflicted on them by their captors, ceased to menstruate.

Charles Darwin (1868) noted that "hard living... retards the period at which animals conceive." When living conditions are hard, the reproductive cycle of women is affected. It's a common belief that underprivileged communities have very high birth rates. This is simply not true. Malnutrition, hardship, and poverty form a lethal triad that frequently results in amenorrhea and infertility. In India, for example, lack of proper birth control does cause great population growth, but the hardships endured by the homeless and poor do take their toll on menstrual health.

Normal menstrual function occurs when a woman is living a healthy, balanced, and contented life. This was certainly not the case for prisoners in Nazi war camps, and it is not the case for any woman who has unnecessary cruelty and hardship inflicted on her. It is unlikely that the hypothalamus will function normally when it is impacted by such intense emotional and physical stress.

General Poor Health and Illness

Sarah was fit and athletic during high school and college, but when she went to work in the city her lifestyle changed. She ate poorly, drank a little too much after work with her colleagues, and stopped getting fresh air and exercise. Every month or so she caught some kind of cold or illness and her periods became light and infrequent.

One of the most common causes of both primary and secondary amenorrhea is general poor health. If you live and eat unhealthily, are stressed or anxious, or indulge to excess in addictions that are toxic for the body, such as smoking, alcohol, or drugs, not only will your health be poor due to a weakened immune system, but menstrual dysfunction is very likely.

Amenorrhea can also occur during times of disease and illness. In response to the stress and energy drain placed on the body by the illness, the reproductive cycle switches off to conserve energy needed for healing. Many women may experience absent or infrequent menses. Even a heavy cold can cause a disruption in the menstrual routine. Usually, periods return when full health is recovered. In cases of serious illness, however, such as kidney or liver failure, cystic fibrosis, diabetes, pituitary or ovarian tumors, or colitis, amenorrhea may be a long-term condition or become permanent. Also, in times of acute infection, like that of pneumonia, the adrenal hormonal response that is triggered to fight the infection may alter the menstrual cycle. Women with HIV, which causes problems with the pituitary gland and low estrogen production, also have noted complaints about amenorrhea.

Some forms of brain damage, such as cerebral palsy, will affect the parts of the brain needed to orchestrate menstruation, and a sharp blow or injury to the head can have a similar effect. Tumors in the hypothalamus or pituitary gland can also often cause so much damage that the glands cannot secrete their hormones and menses cease.

However severe the illness or disease causing absent menstruation is, amenorrhea is a clear indication that health is poor. Your body is ill in some way, or there is some kind of imbalance in your lifestyle. If you know that you lead an unhealthy lifestyle, are not pursuing a regular program of preventive health care, and have been amenorrheaic for more than three months, you should seek treatment immediately.

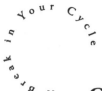

chapter 5

Contraceptives and Amenorrhea

"I never wanted to go on the pill," says Carrie. "I always thought it was so unnatural and unhealthy, but when I went to college I started dating, and it seemed the only sensible thing to do. I couldn't afford to get pregnant. I wanted to go to law school and think about having a family later. Well, I went to law school, got a great career, and got married when I was thirty-one. We put off having a family for a while, as I had to travel so much for my work, but when I got to thirty-four I really didn't want to leave it any longer. I went off the pill and was convinced that after the first month I was pregnant, as no period started. I rushed to the drugstore and bought a home pregnancy kit. It came out negative. I was so disappointed. Months passed by. I don't know how many times I bought a pregnancy kit kind of half hoping that I was pregnant. After eight unbearable months I went to see a doctor, and she told me that some kind of post-pill amenorrhea is quite usual as the system starts to go back to normal. She told me to wait another few months. I did and nothing happened. I'm thirty-five now. I still can't menstruate, and I am sure the pill is to blame. If only I had been warned that this could happen. I'm so angry and unhappy. I had perfectly normal periods before I went on it. I am going to have to see an infertility specialist next week to see if I have become infertile. I feel wretched and helpless."

Most oral contraceptives repress ovulation. They contain progestin (a progesteronelike hormone) and estrogen. These hormones act together to suppress the pituitary hormones FSH and LH, which stimulate the ovary to mature a follicle and release an egg. They also make cervical mucous dry and inhibit the growth of the uterine lining. The dose of estrogen in the pill is far lower than in the past, but some oral contraceptives are more powerful than others. When you go on the pill, your doctor should make you fully aware of what strength of hormone you are taking and how this will impact your cycle. Your past menstrual history and current lifestyle should also be discussed. Some pills do not prevent ovulation at all and just work on the mucous; these may be more suitable for you. For most of us, the low-dose estrogen pill is safe to take, but a very small percentage of women do fail to menstruate when they stop taking the pill.

When you go off the pill your menses should start the next month, although sometimes the hormonal adjustment back to pre-pill days may take up to six months. If it takes any longer you should see a doctor, because some form of hormonal imbalance or other problem has occurred and you need to have it treated and, if possible, corrected.

Why does this happen? Why don't some of us menstruate after being on the pill? For some of us, going on the pill at too early an age is the problem. Your reproductive cycle has not fully established itself, and going on the pill suspends the hormonal axis so that when the pill is withdrawn, amenorrhea occurs. Constantly stopping and starting the pill and taking different dosages may also cause the same problem, as will high levels of stress, overexercise, and a poor diet.

It is easy to understand how Carrie feels. She blames the pill for her amenorrhea and infertility. True, the pill is unnatural because it suppresses a normal female function that should occur every month, but remember that the benefits far outweigh the negatives. The pill makes periods more manageable and gives us tremendous freedom. Unlike our poor ancestors, who were trapped by pregnancy and childbirth for much of their lives, we can prevent unwanted pregnancies and plan our families.

In the early seventies it was believed that the pill caused amenorrhea and that women should take a break from the pill every so often and allow a few months to get it out of the system. We now know that the effect of the pill wears off in a few days. Post-pill amenorrhea that is longer than a few months is not caused by the

A Break in Your Cycle

pill. Similarly, taking the pill is not likely to cause amenorrhea or infertility, because the pill drives the uterus directly, irrespective of the pituitary and the ovaries. What the pill does do, though, is hide problems, hormonal or otherwise, that should perhaps have received treatment earlier, as in Carrie's case. While she was on the pill, her job was very stressful, she traveled a great deal, and she dieted constantly to maintain her sylphlike figure. Had she not been on the pill, her periods may well have stopped several years earlier and alerted her to the fact that she was placing too much stress on her body. She could have sought treatment at a younger age so that starting a family would not have been such a traumatic, anxious time for her.

Some women find that when taking the pill they stop menstruating. This is called pill amenorrhea. Pill amenorrhea is just an exaggeration of what most of us notice when we go on the pill: lighter periods. The progesterone in the pill stops the endometrium from getting too thick, and in some cases the lining is so minimal that menses will become absent or very, very light.

Depo-Provera is a contraceptive injection that also often causes secondary amenorrhea. The medication, given every three months, inhibits pituitary-releasing functions and thereby suppresses ovarian production of estrogen. This hormonal imbalance results in atrophy of the uterine lining, and the majority of women on this medication do become amenorrheaic. Depo-Provera has been used for more than twenty years in many countries around the world, and is almost 100 percent effective in preventing pregnancy. Approved by medical boards for use in the United States, the medication is considered to be safe and to have no harmful side effects or to influence future fertility.

Summary

Amenorrhea is not caused by contraceptive methods. The pill is not dangerous or harmful when it is taken at the correct dose for you. If, however, you are under great stress, suffer from eating disorders, or exercise excessively, or if there is an underlying disease process at work in your body, the contraceptive will mask a hormonal balance or other serious problem. Once you stop taking the pill it will leave your system completely in a few days, but the underlying reason for post-pill menstrual dysfunction, previously hidden by the pill, will not go away until the cause is discovered and treatment is sought.

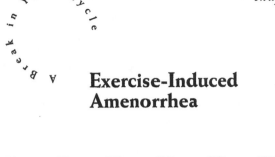

chapter 6

Exercise-Induced Amenorrhea

WOMEN ARE NOW ACTIVE PARTICIPANTS IN COMPETI-
tive and recreational physical activity. There is still great uncertainty,
though, regarding the effect of intense physical activity on our
reproductive system. As more of us participate in exercise and
sports, and training programs become more strenuous, physicians
are seeing an increase in complaints of menstrual cycle disturbances.
Soranus of Ephesus, in the first century AD, mentioned in his treatise "On the Diseases of Women" that "amenorrhea is frequently observed in the youthful, the aged, the pregnant, in singers and those
who take too much exercise." Recent studies prove that if intense
training is begun before puberty, menarche is delayed, and if it begins after menarche, secondary amenorrhea is very common.

Absent or irregular menstruation, intermenstrual bleeding, thinning of the bones, abnormal growth of the uterine lining, and infertility are some of the clinical effects of excessive exercise. The
nature and severity of the symptoms depend on a number of vari-
ables, such as the type of training, its intensity and duration, weekly
mileage, and the rate of progression of the training program.

Menstrual dysfunction is a problem that affects many female athletes, especially those involved in high-intensity and weight-con-
scious sports. Researchers who examined the menstrual cycle of two
hundred runners found that elite runners who ran up to eighty
miles a week were at the greatest risk of developing amenorrhea
(Hetland, et al 1993). Whereas approximately 5 percent of American
women have three or fewer periods a year, in female athletes this
percentage rises to 50 percent. A study by Johnson and Whitaker
published in *The First Aider* in 1997 showed amenorrhea affected 50

percent of competitive runners, 44 percent of ballet dancers, 25 percent of noncompetitive runners, and 12 percent of cyclists, gymnasts, and swimmers.

Low to moderate exercise, say running fifteen to twenty miles a week, does not seem to alter the cycle greatly, but anything more than this becomes borderline and will more than likely result in menstrual abnormalities. Even recreational joggers demonstrate poor follicular development, decreased estrogen and progesterone secretion, and absent ovulation.

More and more women are making exercise and fitness a part of their lives. This is a very positive development. What is not such a positive step forward, however, is the sacrifice of menstrual health in order to pursue ever more exhausting and demanding training schedules.

Doctors are still, in some cases, not expressing enough concern about amenorrhea, and are assuring athletes that eventually normal menses will return. The incorrect belief is that amenorrhea and being an athlete go together. This is a dangerous assumption to make. Athletic amenorrhea is a potentially serious problem. It is associated with hormonal abnormalities that can lead to serious clinical consequences, such as increased incidence of stress fractures, infertility, and loss of bone density. In the words of Dr. Carol Otis, Chairperson of the American College of Sports Medicine Ad Hoc Task Force of Women's Issues in Sports Medicine, "Up until about the early 1980s, most of us regarded amenorrhea as a relatively benign condition and something that was a consequence of training.... Amenorrhea is a symptom of something going wrong. It is not a natural response of the female body to training. It is an indication of a potentially serious clinical problem." (Skolnick 1993).

Athletic amenorrhea is not fully understood yet, but it is believed to be the result of hypothalamic dysfunction, which, as I have explained earlier, results in dysfunction throughout the entire hormonal axis system. A number of theories are circulating at present about why female athletes are more prone to hypothalamic amenorrhea than others. One of these is the relation of low body weight to menstrual dysfunction.

A Break in Your Cycle

Low Body Weight

"When I won my scholarship to a London ballet school," says Rebecca, an ex-dancer, "I was thrilled. But I never really thought it through—the extreme discipline and need for a slim physique. When I entered the school I was about one hundred and ten pounds at a height of four feet six inches, and I was the heaviest girl in my class. It was the weekly weigh-ins that terrified me. They were on Mondays so I would not eat for the entire weekend before. I went on a strict diet. You can't imagine my delight when I eventually weighed in at just over ninety pounds. I didn't mind that my periods had stopped; it was a small price to pay for the satisfaction being thin gave me. From being the one nobody noticed, I was suddenly offered a place in the company. That's when the real problems began. Keeping my weight down just wasn't easy anymore without the school discipline and routine. The pounds piled back on. I got desperate and tried everything I could, but I guess my body is just not happy being that thin. It got to the point where I collapsed in rehearsals one day due to laxative abuse, and ever since then I just can't get my strength back anymore. I'm working in advertising now. Sometimes I really miss the dancing, but all that dieting has damaged my health. I tire easily and still haven't got my periods back."

Joanna is an eighteen-year-old scholarship student of ballet. She trains for six to seven hours a day and works in the evening as a waitress. For the last two months she has been inducing vomiting on a regular basis in order to maintain her weight of ninety pounds at a height of five feet three inches. Her diet consists of the occasional orange, diet sodas, and chewing gum. She has never had a menstrual period.

Nina is a twenty-two-year-old member of a ballet company. She started to menstruate when she was fourteen and then went into serious dance training when she was fifteen. She has not menstruated for the last six years. Her weight at the date of her last period was about one hundred and ten pounds. She now weighs ninety-five pounds and is five feet six inches tall.

Amanda is a competitive runner. She has irregular periods and notices that whenever she falls below hundred pounds she becomes amenorrheaic.

During puberty, menses first occur when body fat content rises above 17 percent and cease when it falls below 12 percent. When body fat is too low to support a baby, the body is in a state of stress because it is malnourished, and so the hypothalamus does not send out signals to orchestrate the menstrual cycle. Many athletes, dancers, and gymnasts are below the twelve percent body fat threshold, and as a result they are amenorrheaic. Competitive female athletes often have 50 percent less body fat than nonexercisers. Usually when a woman is around a hundred pounds, her reproductive cycle shuts down, but the critical fat level is different for every woman, and sometimes when fat is replaced by muscle (with swimmers, for example) the body fat loss may be hard to detect.

Exercise-induced amenorrhea is most frequently seen in ballet dancers, skaters, gymnasts, and long distance runners. These athletes claim that an extremely low body fat makes training easier and is aesthetically more pleasing. The five-foot five-inch dancer who weighs in at ninety-eight pounds and is desperate to lose another seven so that she can audition for a ballet company would not be an unusual case. Despite looking desperately frail, she will still consider herself to be overweight. This may seem illogical, but a dancer is a victim of her profession. As unhealthy as it may sound, the requirement of most ballet companies is for thin—very thin— dancers. An extra five pounds could cost a young dancer a place in the company.

The pressure to be lean and light in some sports encourages eating disorders and poor nutrition as misguided attempts to reduce weight. These conditions are associated with amenorrhea. An inadequate energy supply, due to lack of protein and insufficient vitamins and minerals, plus a heavy training schedule, means that the period just cannot survive. For athletes, the combination of heavy training with inadequate food intake, low caloric input, and high caloric expenditure will result in primary and secondary amenorrhea and menstrual disturbances.

In the cases that opened this section, the fatness level relates to whether menstruation occurs or not. If Nina and Amanda fall below the necessary body fat requirement, their periods will either become irregular or stop altogether. In the case of Joanna, there is not enough body fat in the first place for her to start menstruating. Our bodies need a certain percentage of fat to maintain the reproductive cycle, and ultimately, to support pregnancy. If we deplete these energy stores we disrupt the menstrual cycle.

Athletic Training

When Louise had to take three months off from ballet due to a groin injury, she menstruated for the first time. Her weight did not change much from the ninety-five pounds she was before the injury occurred.

Victoria is a busy skiing instructor. She only seems to menstruate when she takes a vacation from her teaching schedule. Her weight does not alter significantly when she is on vacation.

While body fat and body weight do play a role in menstrual dysfunction, the body fat explanation does not account for cases like those of ballet dancers who resume their periods with no change in body weight but who are forced to rest because of injury. Their amenorrhea returns when the training returns.

Here the absence of menstrual bleeding seems to be related in some way to the training schedule of the athlete and not so much to body fat.

The high incidence of amenorrhea during training is well documented, and it is related in some way to the stress placed on the body by sustained physical exertion over long periods of time. Experts such as Dr. P. T. Ellison, a Harvard anthropologist, have shown that energy expenditure is more likely to cause periods to stop than weight loss. Although increased training often goes hand in hand with a reduction in body fat, the indications are that an intense training schedule does alter the menstrual cycle regardless of body fat. The whole area is underresearched and much is still to be learned, but we do know that the fabled "runner's high" (the body's own morphinelike painkiller), which is produced after a certain amount of aerobic training, can interfere with normal hypothalamic function. Also, the psychological and emotional stresses of strenuous exercise are associated with an increase in cortisol (an adrenal stress hormone), which also affects the hypothalamus. In the amenorrheaic athlete, the adrenal gland may be secreting cortisol at near maximum levels even at rest. With so many factors fighting against them, the ovaries don't really stand much of a chance.

Athletic amenorrhea occurs when the stress of intense training causes dysfunction in the hypothalamus, which leads to progressive dysfunction through the entire hormonal axis system. Running is a good example to illustrate how intense exercise can impact your menstrual cycles. If you run more than thirty or so miles a week, you cause a rise in beta-endorphins. These "feel good" hormones give you a "high," a pleasurable feeling of well-being, but they also upset the hypothalamic-pituitary-ovarian axis by suppressing the release of FSH and LH from the pituitary gland, causing decreased ovarian estrogen secretion. With insufficient estrogen, shedding of the uterine lining in menstruation cannot occur. Your exercise routine is also releasing cortisol from the adrenal gland, which interferes with the release of FSH and LH, too.

The Professional Athlete

Linda, thirty-five, had a glorious career as a principal dancer. From the age of five she lived, breathed, and devoted herself to dance. When she became thirty-five, her contract with the company was terminated, and she went back to college. She met Paul, within a year they were married, and they have since tried unsuccessfully to start a family. Linda was amenorrheaic for most of her dancing years, and in the last few years has had only a few irregular periods. She has undergone expensive medical testing by doctors and visited private clinics to try to rectify her amenorrhea and apparent infertility.

Great physical demands and emotional pressures are placed on athletes and performers today. The expectation of physical excellence is higher than ever. More and more women are entering sport-related professions. Training regimens are getting more and more intense, and coaching begins at an earlier and earlier age. The pressure to win, succeed, and beat the odds has become so competitive that it is hard to keep a sense of perspective and maintain a healthy, balanced life alongside the athletic career. Even winning once is not enough; the need to win again and again and again, to push the body harder and harder, is often all that an athlete, after a lifetime dedicated to a craft, knows how to do.

Women who are amenorrheaic because of overexercise often resemble anorexics in their absent periods, their desire to be in control of their bodies, their passion about what they do, and their relentless pursuit of an ideal body form. There are, however, distinctions between the true anorexic and many professional athletes. The anorexic will not consider herself underweight and will not care about her poor physical condition, whereas an athlete or a dancer will often be able to see that there is a problem and will do something about it when it is affecting performance.

Many women who engage in exercise tend to develop varying degrees of anorexic reaction although they will not be anorexic as such. The reaction develops unconsciously as the woman strives for perfection in her art or her sport, but she will not generally develop the emotional and psychological problems associated with eating disorders.

For various reasons, when a woman is in intense training and/or her body reaches a critically low fat level, her ability to produce estrogen is affected. Estrogen is the important hormone in the production of the uterine lining each month and is related to fat and ovarian production and the production of necessary bone tissue. Without any of these systems working properly, the woman will not menstruate. If the amenorrhea has continued for a very long period of time, as in Linda's case, the amenorrhea may not reverse itself back to normal menstrual function, even after the vigorous training has stopped.

Physicians are only just becoming more concerned about the menstrual health of female athletes. The term used to describe the problem is called the "Female Athlete Triad." This refers to the triad of separate but interrelated disorders observed in adolescent and young adult women athletes, namely disordered eating, amenorrhea, and osteoporosis. The term may be new but the problem is not. Female athletes have come forward with these complaints for many years, but little attention has been paid to them. It is time for the medical profession to pay more attention to this new epidemic and for recognition, treatment, and prevention to be more readily available.

Athletes, gymnasts, skaters, and dancers undertake a training program because, in most cases, this is their chosen vocation and what they want to devote their lives to. Their professions require them to push their bodies to extraordinary limits. Discipline, hard work, and a certain amount of suffering are necessary if they want to excel. This may be true, but athlete or not, any woman who is a heavy exerciser, who is a poor eater, and who does not have a menstrual cycle should consult a physician. Later in life when the training ceases and the menses do not return, emotional problems can occur. It is more natural and healthy for women who want to bear children to have a menstrual cycle. A woman doesn't need to be amenorrheaic to be a better athlete.

The Exercise Addict

Katie, twenty-seven, is a bundle of energy. She works for an advertising company by day, but by night she is an aerobics instructor. She usually teaches one or two classes a night and follows that with her own training, which includes forty-five minutes on the stair-stepping machine and at least an hour of weights. If she misses her training or her classes she finds herself getting extremely agitated. "I don't know," she says, "it's just something I have to do. If I don't, I feel so guilty and useless. My exercise routine makes me feel that I have achieved something every day. It makes me feel better about myself. I used to train four times week but now I need a daily fix.

Mary's daily jog is between four and six miles. Occasionally she will miss a day or two but she feels uncomfortable and guilty about it. Since she started taking jogging seriously and running races, she has noticed that she skips periods. Absent menses have not bothered her; she says being amenorrheaic actually makes running easier because her stamina has improved.

"I know that I'm obsessed about running" says Miranda, thirty-nine. "But if I don't run, I don't feel that I am living." Miranda is thin and wiry looking with bandages on her knees and dark circles around her eyes. Despite being extremely fit, she does not look like a picture of health. She runs an average of eight to ten miles a day and has competed successfully in marathons all over the country. She has been amenorrheaic for four years.

As equally disturbing as the high incidence of amenorrhea in female athletes is the occurrence of amenorrhea among women who are not professional athletes but who are obsessed with exercise.

These women choose to pursue a grueling exercise regimen alongside their other commitments, work, and family. Exercise "fix" is exactly how Katie's devotion to her exercise routine should be described. It has gone from being a pleasurable activity to a compulsion, and there are an alarming number of women like her, many of whom, because their symptoms are milder than Katie's, are not even aware that they are becoming addicted. Others, like Miranda, know that their devotion to exercise is abnormal but they can't change.

A love of physical movement and participation in sports and exercise can enrich a person's life. It is a well-known and researched fact that the integration of an exercise program into your weekly schedule makes you feel and look better, increases your energy levels, wards off disease, and lengthens the life span. The huge interest in health and fitness of the last few decades has encouraged people to take better care of themselves, and this is a very positive development. A small minority of women, however, have become addicted to the feeling of well-being that exercises offers.

The famous "runner's high," which can be achieved after about thirty minutes of aerobic exercise, has been described in religious terminology, equating it to a spiritual awakening. Exercise has for some become the cure for all evils. Yet a woman who chooses to exercise for several hours a day and who is not a professional athlete is overdoing a good thing and is becoming addicted. Any addiction is harmful if it starts to become an obsession. For true athletes, the exercise complements their lives; for exercise victims, exercise is their life and literally runs it.

For those who have never heard of the term, exercise addiction is a frame of mind that enables someone to pursue an exercise program for long periods of time. Running is the example that most often springs to mind, but all aerobic sports are based on continued movement for increasing amounts of time. Explanations include the "runner's high" and the possibility of replacing negative addictions, such as smoking, drugs, and alcohol, with something positive. Having experienced the physical and psychological advantages of exercise, some people think they can never get enough. If one workout makes them feel so good, why not do another and another?

Women who feel alienated, who lack confidence in themselves for some reason, or who are facing crisis points in their lives are especially vulnerable to exercise addiction. Training becomes the only thing that can make them feel right, so they pursue it to extremes. An addiction to fitness is hard to criticize because it is something that society approves of in this age of health, fitness, and well-being. There is, as a result, very little help available for sufferers, even though their condition is just as potentially dangerous an addiction as drugs and alcohol when taken to extremes. An overexercised, exhausted body leads to fatigue and depression. The stress of the exercise regimen causes hypothalamic malfunction and amenorrhea. Injuries are not allowed to heal, the muscles and joints are strained to the limits, the body's metabolism is confused, and the major organs are forced to work overtime, until they eventually give up and refuse to cooperate.

Exercise is only good for you if it is not taken to extremes. It is important to have some discipline and to stick to an exercise plan, but if you find yourself becoming agitated if for a few days you have to ease up, or if you exercise even when you are exhausted or injured, then you are becoming addicted.

A clear warning sign of overexercise is the absence of menses. If you are amenorrheaic you have reached a stage where your exercise program has become more important than your health and physical well-being. When you need a workout every day, even if you have injuries, your exercise obsession has become potentially life-threatening.

When a woman faces difficulties in her life and lacks confidence in herself, she can be tempted to become compulsive, to keep on running instead of facing issues. In actuality, that is the very time that she should be slowing down the pace a little and dealing with what life has presented her—not in a negative, self-destructive, compulsive way, but in a positive, self-affirming, and balanced manner.

If you notice that you have not had a period for six months and you are training and dieting heavily, you should take this warning sign from your body very seriously. Unless positive lifestyle changes are made and priorities reassessed, you will almost certainly have to face distressing health complications and problems in the future.

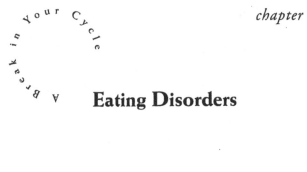

chapter 7

Eating Disorders

FEW OF US CAN DENY THAT AT SOME POINT IN OUR LIVES we have been concerned about our weight and considered dieting. You may be among the fortunate few who never have to worry about your body weight, but more likely you belong to the great majority of us who have to struggle with our weight and watch our food intake. We enjoy eating, but we feel guilty whenever we indulge. "I'll just eat a little less tomorrow and do an extra step class this week," we say to ourselves unconvincingly.

Women and food. What a complicated love-hate relationship we have with it! It is the comforter, the nurturer, a way of giving and receiving affection, a way of sharing, and—if you believe the saying "you are what you eat"—a way of living. If it is so many wonderful things, why is it also something that causes fear, guilt, resentment, and shame? Why do we have this complex relationship with food? Because often our need for food is not physical but emotional hunger. Instead of being angry we eat, instead of feeling lonely we eat, instead of feeling sad we comfort ourselves with food. We use food to avoid addressing unresolved emotional issues.

In our quest for a sense of self, many of us stumble when it comes to food. Overcoming our obsession with food and coming to terms with our body weight is a major rite of passage for many women. Only when we can say we are in control of our eating and have a balanced healthy body image can we satisfy the real inner hunger for a fulfilling relationship with ourselves, others, and society. If we cannot do this, we will be condemned to years of guilt, anxiety, dieting, and food obsession.

Cultural Standards of Beauty

It is during vulnerable times in our lives, when confusion about what we really want in life becomes entangled with confusion about food, that we are most likely to develop disordered eating habits. Eating disorders, because of the stress they place on the body's digestive system and the inadequate nutritional status of the body, do cause amenorrhea. Some five million American women suffer from eating disorders, ranging from compulsive dieting to compulsive eating, anorexia, and bulimia. Billions and billions of dollars are spent every year on ways to lose weight.

Society's constant emphasis on beauty, thinness, and fashion is partly to blame here. We are living in a century that has been obsessed with the ideal of thinness ever since Twiggy (ninety-two pounds and five feet seven inches) became what women foolishly aspired to look like thirty years ago, regardless of body type and shape. The incredibly thin fashion models who parade the world's catwalks are sylphlike icons. For the great majority of us, this quite simply is an impossible ideal to attain. We are all born with different body types. Some are more naturally slender than others, and no amount of dieting will change body shape. Yet despite this, women throughout the ages have tried to mold and change their body shape, and have tortured themselves to conform to the ever changing body ideal of current fashion trends. Think, for instance, of the barbaric corsets of the eighteenth and nineteenth century, designed to reduce a woman's waist to eighteen inches so it could be small enough for a man to hold in both his hands.

In prehistoric societies, chunky women were "in." Being obese with large pendulous breasts was considered a sign of beauty. Now, centuries later, we have gradually "progressed" to the opposite end of the spectrum. Being thin is "in." So "in" that it is often all young girls care about in their desire to look like the fashion trendsetters and celebrity "role models." Being thin is more highly valued than career, health, marriage, and family, and in a recent survey being fat was feared by young girls more than nuclear war or cancer.

Neither the obese nor the thin beauty standard is a healthy role model; somewhere in between would be healthy. There are signs that things are changing and role models are emerging who look strong, healthy, and toned without looking malnourished, but we still have a long way to go before the famous saying, "You can never be too rich or too thin" becomes less of a socially accepted norm.

You *can* be too thin—far too thin—to menstruate. In the absence of disease or physical abnormality, failure to menstruate is frequently linked to malnutrition and low body fat. If your body fat falls below a certain percent, the hypothalamus—reacting to the stress your body is in—malfunctions and ovulation will cease. This is a protective measure on the body's part. It senses that at this low weight you wouldn't be physically able to handle the stress and nutrient drain of pregnancy.

The great majority of us do not have serious eating disorders, smoke or drink to excess, or use illegal substances; we just develop poor eating habits that do not supply our body with the necessary nutrients. Some of us diet too much and become preoccupied with staying thin in an attempt to measure up to society's thin beauty standard. We develop a disordered attitude toward eating, fearing fat as if it were a dangerous disease. If we're lucky, our periods will not stop and we will not put our health at risk before we learn that being thin and wearing a size four pair of jeans is not all that matters—but being healthy and valued for who we are is what matters most.

Low Body Weight

"This is a bit embarrassing really," says Samantha, giggling. She is a very young looking thirty-one-year-old. "But I actually didn't get my first period until I was twenty-five. A real late bloomer! I was such a skinny kid and very proud that I never let my weight go over one hundred pounds. Going to college changed all that though. I suddenly found other things to think and worry about; counting every calorie just got tedious. I got my periods back the year before I graduated."

Until she reached the age of twenty-five, Samantha's diet was inadequate. She was just too thin to menstruate, and so she developed primary amenorrhea. Based on the relation of height and weight at menarche, research reveals that approximately 17 percent of the total body mass must be fat for menstruation to occur, and usually in girls at puberty this critical weight is in the region of one hundred and five pounds.

Samantha began menstruating when her diet improved and she reached one hundred and ten pounds. If she falls below this weight her menses will cease and she will experience secondary amenorrhea. For her periods to start again she would probably have to gain a significantly higher proportion of weight than a hundred and ten pounds; studies also reveal that a greater percentage of body fat, around 22 percent, would now be needed to trigger the system again.

Obesity

"Everybody stares at you when you are fat," says Lisa, thirty-five, discussing her obese teenage years. In the end I used to stop going outside. Everything became too much of an effort; there was never enough room for me. My inner thighs would get scraped and sore from rubbing together when I walked. I'd stay at home all day, and instead of watching my food intake it doubled, then tripled. It was the boredom really. If I - couldn't go out, like everyone else, at least I could enjoy my food, if you can call pizzas and ice cream and chocolate food. My periods stopped when I reached three hundred and twenty pounds. I started to get pains in my chest. If it hadn't been for the patience, love, and devotion of my family I would never have lost nearly two hundred pounds. I would probably have been dead by now. Killed by the thing I love most, food."

Despite society's emphasis on slenderness there are millions of overweight people in the United States. A significant percentage of these are obese. In most cases of obesity, both physical disorders and emotional problems need to be addressed. Many obese women will not ovulate. Too much body fat causes bodily stress, strains the heart, and stops menstruation.

Irregular Eating Habits

Most of us are not obese or painfully thin but are somewhere in between. The greatest threat to menstrual health for us will lie in irregular eating habits due to dieting.

We try to lose a few pounds here and there. One summer we manage to shift ten pounds, only to find the next summer that we have put it back on and added seven more pounds. We decide to go on a strict diet again. It sounds familiar, doesn't it? This kind of disordered eating, or yo-yo dieting, is a lethal cocktail that has the opposite effect of what is intended. The metabolic rate becomes so confused after periods of dieting followed by indulgence that it adopts a starvation mode and slows down. We may be eating less, but our body is holding onto everything it gets for much longer, fearing that starvation might come again. In prehistoric times of famine this is what kept us alive, but our twentieth-century bodies can't distinguish between dieting amid plenty and the threat of famine. If food is restricted, it will go into famine mode. The result is that you eat like a sparrow but you still don't lose weight. Not fair, is it! Fortunately, the long-term effects of disordered eating do not appear to be as severe as once was originally thought. Years of yo-yo dieting do not lower metabolism to the point where you will never be thin. Once a balanced, healthy diet is resumed, your metabolism should eventually return to normal. But, just as obesity and low body fat confuse the body and force it to conserve energy by shutting down the reproductive cycle, yo-yo dieting also stresses the body and has the same effect. The moral of the story: dieting really doesn't work. Sensible, healthy, regular eating does.

An inadequate diet will not only cause general poor health, due to a weakened immune system, but complications such as hypoglycemia and low blood sugar as well. If too much refined sugar is consumed, it gets into the bloodstream too fast, causing the pancreas to overreact. This makes blood-sugar levels plummet, and not only do you become very hungry, but the feedback along the HPO axis is again impacted, causing menstrual dysfunction.

Thyroid problems can also occur if diet is poor. The thyroid is associated with our metabolic rate, the rate at which food is digested and utilized by the body. Sometimes the body will try to conserve energy in a food-deprived state by decreasing thyroid hormone secretion to slow metabolic rate and increase energy. The result is almost always weight gain. Even though you may be eating the same, or less than usual, you will put on weight because food passes through your system at a much slower rate. An underactive thyroid gland can also disrupt normal pituitary ovarian function. If your thyroid gland is not releasing enough thyroid hormone, then your hypothalamus will react by sending signals to the pituitary demanding more thyroid stimulating hormone. Unfortunately, in the process the signals to the pituitary also cause the release of prolactin. Ovulation stops because of high prolactin levels (discussed in Chapter 9), and amenorrhea occurs.

Unhealthy Substances

Maggie began smoking when she was fourteen and soon became addicted. By the age of twenty-eight she was smoking more than sixty cigarettes a day. She became amenorrheaic when she was thirty, and she went into menopause when she was thirty-five.

What we take into our bodies is crucial for a healthy reproductive cycle. An unhealthy diet or unhealthy substances such as too much alcohol, nicotine, caffeine, or drugs will in the long term adversely affect menstruation. Drugs are a major cause of amenorrhea, especially marijuana and heroin. Once these substances get into the bloodstream they influence every cell in the body and inhibit ovulation. Frequently, drug users also have a terrible diet and are underweight, so it is often a combination of malnutrition and drug use that causes amenorrhea.

Smoking has been linked to an increased risk of early menopause and osteoporosis in women. It increases the risk by robbing you of your estrogen as a premenopausal woman. Cigarettes, like alcohol, taken in excess over long periods, do inhibit ovulation.

Anorexia Nervosa

Catherine is the youngest child in a large, wealthy family. She lacks confidence despite the fact that she does very well at school. She is very shy and feels that she never has anything to contribute and that the only way she can gain respect and attention is to please others. She keeps herself scrupulously clean and is very concerned about her weight. She is five foot seven and weighs eighty-five pounds. She says she feels fat if she gets above ninety pounds. Her clothes are baggy and multi-layered, even in summer. She says she always feels cold. She looks older than her nineteen years and her hair is getting very thin. She has no breast development and has never had a menstrual period. She has taken over much of the housework at home because she knows her three younger brothers are too much for her mother to cope with alone. Her father is a successful lawyer, and her mother is an ex-teacher who suffers from depression. Catherine is very worried about her mother and feels that she should be there for her. Catherine jogs every day for nearly two hours and has developed a complicated body-conditioning routine, which she usually performs at night. It includes sit-ups, press-ups, leg raises, and body curls, and the repetitions of each movement are in the hundreds. If she misses or omits any part of her routine she feels anxious and guilty. She never feels hungry but constantly thinks about food. Thinking is about all she will let herself do, though. She hardly ever succumbs to the occasional craving she has for sweets and ice cream. If she does indulge she will induce vomiting, and if that fails she will take huge amounts of laxatives to expel the food from her system.

Food is about the only area of Catherine's life where she feels that she has really succeeded and shown discipline and control. Even though she wanted to be a nurse, her father has decided that she will study law instead. Her diet consists of one apple daily and one bowl of cereal. Sometimes she will omit the fat-free milk from her cereal, and sometimes she will cut down her allotted two hundred cereal flakes to one hundred if she is feeling fat.

Some of us get hopelessly caught up in the quest for slenderness and take it to dangerous extremes. Estimates suggest that as many as eight million people in the United States, many of whom go undetected, could have serious eating disorders. When eating disorders develop, like anorexia nervosa or bulimia nervosa, there are profound psychological problems, and these must first be treated before progress of any sort can be made. Eating disorders have received a great deal of press attention in the last few years as more is being learned about them, and as well-known personalities confess to being sufferers. Karen Carpenter and Princess Diana immediately spring to mind.

Although victims of anorexia nervosa can and do come from all sorts of backgrounds, it does seem to affect a certain type of woman more than others. Hilde Bruch, in her important study on anorexia nervosa, *The Golden Cage* (1987), writes, "New diseases are rare and a disease that selectively befalls the young, rich and beautiful is practically unheard of. But such a disease is affecting the daughters of well-to-do educated and successful families, not only in the United States but in many other affluent countries. The chief symptom is severe starvation leading to a devastating weight loss; 'she looks like the victim of a concentration camp' is not an uncommon description."

Bruch is right; the incidence of anorexia nervosa in young middle- to upper-class females under the age of twenty-five is very high. It can also strike at any socioeconomic level and at any age, but case histories of anorexics do tend to have certain similarities. Families of anorexics are often success-orientated and concerned about how they appear to the rest of the world. Serious problems may exist within the family but they remain hidden from the world, until the anorexic expresses the pain and dysfunction through her body. Frequently there are high expectations for the anorexic child, who is thought to be the perfect daughter. Typically she begins a diet as a form of rebellion when the weight gain of puberty is perceived as excessive. Then, as she adds high activity levels, her body weight drops and amenorrhea occurs. Often anorexics tend to be overachievers, and they value discipline and control. They usually end up socially isolated. Menstruation will cease when body fat is too low, and constipation and abdominal pain is common. There is a preoccupation with food and laxative abuse. Skin becomes dry and yellowish, and soft hair grows on the back and buttocks.

There are degrees of eating dysfunction that cause amenorrhea, from the mild crash diet to the severe anorexia, like Catherine's, which is life-threatening if untreated. Doctors must be able to detect what they are dealing with when a patient complains of amenorrhea. The diagnosis of anorexia is always individual, but often doctors will use guidelines like these:

1. Onset between ages ten and thirty
2. Weight loss of 25 percent or weight 15 percent below normal
    weight for age and height
3. Special attitudes:
   • Denial
   • Distorted body image
   • Unusual hoarding and excessive preoccupation with food
4. At least one of the following:
   • Body hair
   • Yellowish tinge to the skin
   • Overactivity
   • Episodes of overeating
   • Vomiting, which may be self-induced

5. Amenorrhea
6. No known medical illness
7. No other psychiatric disorder
8. Other characteristics:
   • Constipation
   • Low blood pressure
   • Diabetes insipidus

Debate rages about whether anorexia is an illness or a psychological state. Probably a combination of both would be the answer. Anorexics do have severe psychological and emotional problems, but to call the problem a disease is correct in the sense that anorexia plays havoc with the body, causing heart problems, low levels of thyroid hormones, and lack of menstruation. If treatment is not sought, death is more than likely if the starvation continues. An estimated 15 to 20 percent will starve themselves to death.

The media is often a reflection of cultural trends, and if proof was needed of the prevalence of eating disorders in today's society, it would be found here. We have made-for-TV movies, hour-long documentaries, self-help manuals, as-told-to autobiographies, and a new generation of novelists who are attempting to turn the problem into literature. Within the last few years more than a dozen or so highly praised novels have told the story of eating disorder victims, from the onset of the disorder to full-blown hospital scenes. Among the most eminently readable, interesting, accurate, and critically acclaimed in their presentation are:
   • *Holy Anorexia* (Bell 1987)
   • *The Passion of Alice* (Grant 1995)
   • *Eve's Apple* (Rosen 1997)
   • *Life Size* (Shute 1995)
   • *The Kiss* (Harrison 1997)
   • *Hunger Point* (Medoff 1997)

These are to name but a few. Publishers are receiving hundreds of manuscripts on the subject and compete to sign up accounts of life-threatening eating disorders, paying six-figure advances in some cases. Many of the novels are gory, detailed in the description of the disorder and at times unpleasantly realistic. It's hard to believe people want to read about this, but the interesting fact is that they do. The books are selling and well. Why? Interest in the details of someone else's life and our shared fascination for food, dieting, and bodily functions, perhaps? Or maybe the appeal of the novels also lies in the fact that, despite the emphasis on the struggle with the body, there is an element of soul searching in them all. All the heroines strive away from attachment to the flesh and aspire toward spiritual perfection. In these novels we read about real women we can relate to who search for some sort of meaning in their lives; a search that they are prepared to risk their lives for. In that way they almost come across as heroic; but the obviously dangerous and misguided method they chose to "improve" themselves, although fascinating to read about, prevents the problem from ever becoming truly glamorized.

Bulimia

Anne has been a dieter all her life, seesawing between periods of fasting and overindulgence. The first time she made herself sick was after her eighteenth birthday dinner. She had eaten too much and, remembering something she had read in a magazine, she stuck her fingers down her throat and tried to vomit. It really hurt, but eventually after thirty minutes of gagging she brought the whole meal up. It seemed the ideal solution. She could eat but not gain any weight. Soon she was vomiting on a regular basis and after six months could even bring up food by simply pressing on her stomach. The only trouble was that she had to consume larger and larger amounts in order to vomit, and most evenings she would work her way through about four normal meals. She would drink lots of liquids to make vomiting easier and would always start her binge with a glass of tomato juice so she could tell when she saw it again in her vomit that all the food had been expelled.

Currently Anne is amenorrheaic. Her once busy social life has disappeared and her plans for college have been postponed. She puts all her energy and time into vomiting, and what had once seemed like relief has now become a nightmarish existence that she is hopelessly addicted to. Her condition is physically, financially, and mentally draining. The tragedy is that although she knows her behavior is abnormal, she feels powerless to do anything about it.

Like anorexia, the related disorder bulimia nervosa is on the increase. Often victims of eating disorders suffer from a combination of both anorexia and bulimia and indulge in episodes of both. Bulimia, like anorexia, affects hypothalamic function, stresses the body, inhibits menstruation, and is very dangerous. It is a syndrome marked by episodes of binge eating followed by self-induced vomiting, fasting, or the use of laxatives. Shoplifting and depression are also common as the disorder begins to take over the sufferer's life in every way. Like anorexia, the problems associated with bulimia are dysfunction of the body mechanisms regulated by the hypothalamus: appetite, thirst, water conservation, temperature, balance, sleep, and the reproductive cycle.

Eating disorders do require urgent treatment because of the dangerous stress they place the body in. When chronic anorexia, vomiting, or obesity are the case it is the whole person who needs to be treated and not just the body. There is little point in treating the physical problems without proper psychiatric guidance and care. The resumption of menstruation may be a sign that the body is getting well, but in order for the recovery to be complete emotional health also needs to be restored. This is not always easy. Patients with eating disorders are among the most difficult to treat. Food and appearance have become about the only area in their lives where they feel that they have control, and any attempt by others to invade this private space will be vigorously rejected. They are frequently defensive, paranoid, and vindictive toward those trying to treat them, but at the same time they are desperately sensitive and needy of attention and understanding. This short fictional scenario illustrates the common experience:

"Sally, I have a picture I want you to look at for me," the doctor says.

What now, I wonder. More photographs of me as a chubby baby, me wrestling with my dog, me with my parents looking shabby, me looking hideous in a swimsuit. Can't they understand that I don't want to see those pictures from my past? I was a different person then—fleshy, needy, and heavy.

I look down at my fingernails and pick at the loose skin until it bleeds. The doctor clears his throat and the social worker tries to catch my eye. I look away from her at the wall and grin, enjoying the embarrassment I am causing. Well, what do they expect? I never asked to be here with these bloated strangers who want to regulate my food intake.

The doctor places a picture in my lap. It has the number 36b written on the top left-hand corner. It is a picture of a young woman photographed from the front, back, and side. She is naked and black slashes cover her eyes and her genitals. I gasp; for once the doctor has shown me something that captures my interest. I can admire this woman. She is thin, very, very thin. I feel a tinge of jealousy, but it is soon replaced with awe. This woman has surpassed rotting flesh—she is bone. Her knee and elbow joints look huge and I have never seen such long arms. It even looks as if she has achieved what I thought impossible—her thighs just have skin and no flesh at all on them. I am filled with deep respect and veneration. I can see every one of her ribs as they strain beneath the skin on her chest. Every vertebrae in her back stands out sharp, pure, and beautiful. Her face is caved in.

I did not realize that you could be that thin and still alive. She surely has reached ultimate perfection: a living skeleton. With every fiber of my being I long to be like her. From now on my goals will be reset, my food intake halved to just one apple daily, my exercise regimen doubled. With this vision before me I can transcend everything now. This picture will be my obsession, my ideal, my meaning.

I feel a tear forming in my eye and resent the presence of the doctor and the social worker intruding upon my private rapture.

"Do you see yourself when you see that picture?" asks the doctor.

"No I have a long way to go before I can be that perfect," I answer.

The doctor rubs his forehead. The social worker shifts uncomfortably from one foot to the other. She strokes my cheek but I move away fast. She tries to take the picture from me but I won't let her have it. A terrible tiredness comes over me and

I hug the picture to my chest like a nursing baby. The doctor says nothing; the social worker scribbles in her notebook.

They depart from the room. My eyes fill with tears and I am sure that I have done something wrong again. Just like I failed my parents, my school, and myself. I'm bad, I know, but I can't seem to help it. Usually I don't care when everybody goes away. I want them to let me be, but this time I really don't want to be left alone with this picture.

The recovery of an anorexic or bulimic in treatment will eventually lie in her own hands. The will to live must come from herself, but the role family, friends, and doctors play in patiently being there for her, understanding her, and caring for her both physically and emotionally—by helping her rebuild her shattered self-confidence—is vital and could mean the difference between life and death.

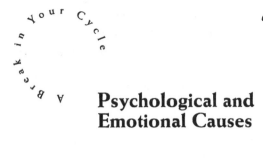
Psychological and Emotional Causes

THE LINK BETWEEN WHAT WE THINK AND HOW WE FEEL has been well documented. We now know that a healthy mind encourages a healthy body and that a state of intense depression or confusion can manifest itself physically in poor health or disease. This chapter will examine how psychological or emotional states, caused either by a stressful situation or by a negative mindset, influence the menstrual cycle.

So much of our thinking, our feeling, and our behavior is unconscious. We do a thing over and over again until we don't need to consciously think about it anymore. For many of us, brushing teeth and hair, and applying creams, lotions, and makeup is just part of a routine that requires little thought. Once something has been learned, conscious thought about it is reduced to a minimum. Patterns are conditioned into our bodies, programming us to act in a certain way. Sometimes we get nervous about a situation that is not, in most cases, dangerous simply because we have become used to feeling anxious about it. Examples include leaving home, dating a new boyfriend, getting married, or taking a driving exam. The mind, because of conditioning, cannot tell the difference anymore between events that are really threatening, and events that have become dangerous in thought alone.

Previous conditioning will affect how our minds work. The attitudes of role models, parents, and the society we have been born into are very influential. The negative responses of society in general toward menstruation have certainly conditioned the way many women feel about it. You may recall the day of your first period. Everybody, including you, was perhaps too embarrassed or confused to discuss it openly. The pain and discomfort that often accompanies menstruation, coupled with this negative mindset, meant that many of us were conditioned to believe that menstruation is indeed a "curse," when it is not.

If menstruation signals womanhood but is perceived as also somehow shameful, dirty, and revolting, how are we then to perceive ourselves—as dirty and revolting too?

It is interesting to consider how very different many women's perceptions of themselves would have been if, instead of keeping menarche a big, nasty secret, the family celebrated it as if it were an important rite of passage, an exciting turning point in a woman's life. Unfortunately, though, like Pavlov's dogs, we have become conditioned. If we have grown up absorbing negative messages about being a female, and if menstruation is the mark of womanhood, then we may, as a result, decide unconsciously that we want no part of menstruation or anything else to do with being a woman. This kind of denial will cause emotional stress.

Psychological and emotional stress can suppress the menstrual function. How we think and feel does impact the menstrual cycle. Our menstrual clock is regulated by the hypothalamus at the base of the brain and stimulated by the impulses of our conscious thoughts and actions. If these stimulations are of a sufficient intensity they can alter the normal menstrual cycle. Amenorrhea is associated with anxiety, depression, loneliness, and fear. The story of St. Wilgefortis illustrates that it can also be connected with the unconscious stress of feeling negative about being a woman.

> St. Wilgefortis, the crucified anorexic saint, became a symbol of women who liberated themselves from female problems. She also became a protectress of women with sexual problems and problems with childbirth. She lived around the year 1000 and was the seventh daughter of the king of Portugal. She made a vow of virginity to become a nun but was confronted with an arranged marriage. Her response was to find deliverance in intense prayer and fasting. Her periods stopped, she looked gaunt and ill, and she grew body hair. When her intended, the king of Sicily, saw his bride, he was revolted and changed his mind, backing out of the marriage. Wilgefortis' father was furious and took the drastic step of having her crucified. In the centuries that followed legend spread around this

A Break in Your Cycle

persecuted girl, probably because there were others like her. Any woman who hated her husband or dreaded the thought of an arranged marriage prayed to Wilgefortis. In England she became known as St. Uncumber because she could help women who prayed to uncumber themselves of their hus- bands.

Conditioned attitudes about the helplessness of women can create feelings of weakness, inferiority, and loss of control over your life. Wilgefortis certainly felt that as a woman she had very little choice about how she would lead her life. Like her, you may have a negative picture of the feminine, and your absent periods may reveal an unconscious resistance or resentment of being female. Menstruation may remind you of female helplessness and inferiority. Society seems to value the male qualities of leadership, drive, ambition, and material gain, so becoming amenorrheaic may make you feel strong and in control, less like the stereotypical, dependent, compliant woman.

The retreat into a more masculine guise could be related in some way to an anxiety about female development in today's world. The amenorrheaic stance may represent a massive confusion of identity, an expression of our longing to escape from the traditional idea of what it is to be a woman, as we try to understand the role of women in an ever-changing world. In some ways it does reveal how strong our wish is to attain more power and authority alongside men, but it also expresses how uncertain we are of our ability as women to do so. We mistakenly think that the only way to gain more power is to be more masculine, and as a result we neglect our incredible potential as women to attain power.

Amenorrhea could also signify an unconscious fear of men and difficulty with relationships. As long as Wilgefortis' body was unattractive, lacking basic female functions, she knew she was safe from the king of Sicily. Relationships are important for a healthy and fulfilled life, but they are not always easy. Sometimes when a woman has problems relating intimately to others, both sexually and nonsexually, this will affect the reproductive organs of sexuality, creation, and relationship. The failure to build successful relationships, with both men and women, could be due to any number of reasons—lack of self-confidence, disappointment with past relationships, fear of dependency, and so on—but whatever the reason, when bonding with others does not occur there will be anxiety. Anxiety, loneliness, and isolation are stressful, and stress inhibits menstrual function.

In the medieval age, Wilgefortis' anorexic stance was explained as a woman's response to the fear of sexuality, marriage, and the trauma of childbirth. Her fasting was interpreted as a morbid fear of fat that indicated a morbid fear of her future as an adult and as a sexually mature woman. Menstruation signals becoming a mature woman, and as long as there are no periods, the childlike fantasy can be maintained. Today a woman who remains persistently amenorrheaic due to an eating disorder may be frightened of growing up, of becoming independent, of losing parental care and protection of making decisions, and of forming adult relationships.

Amenorrhea is a complex physical condition, and the emotions that contribute to its development are equally complex, buried so deeply within each individual's unconscious and the unconscious of the collective feminine. Menstruation is a crucial stage in female self-development: a time for a woman to truly begin to find a sense of identity in a world where she can at last accept, or reject, the challenge of becoming more than the traditional idea of the feminine. For some of us this is an exciting opportunity. For others it represents a time of great uncertainty, anguish, and confusion. We want to move forward but we don't know how. We want to relate to others but lack the confidence to do so. We think we are in control, but our crisis of identity reveals itself in our poor health and amenorrhea.

If a woman is denying—or is repelled by—menstruation, she is denying and is repelled by a part of herself. This rejection of the self can only result in feelings of helplessness and loss of control. Women who feel in control of their lives can cope with and accept change (in fact, they thrive on it). Helplessness, however, is characterized by a decreased motivation to encounter life's difficulties and to embrace change. Amenorrhea may have started as an unconscious defense mechanism, a way to feel stronger or a way to cope with or avoid change, but it can actually make the situation worse. It can contribute toward the creation of a negative mindset that makes it hard to appreciate that you can do anything right. It could be the start of a downward spiral of insecurity, self-loathing, depression, isolation, and illness.

A Break in Your Cycle

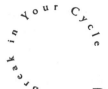

chapter 9

Problems with the Pituitary, Thyroid, Adrenal, and Ovarian Glands

Problems with the Pituitary Gland

A fairly common cause of amenorrhea is overproduction of the hormone prolactin by the pituitary gland. When this happens it is called hyperprolactinemic amenorrhea.

Prolactin is the hormone that promotes lactation. Prolactin prepares the breast to give milk, and levels will go up during pregnancy and after delivery to produce milk for the baby. During pregnancy high levels of estrogen cause the prolactin-making cells of the pituitary, called lactotrophs, to increase. The result is that the pituitary gland expands, prolactin production increases, and ovulation stops. During breast-feeding a woman needs all the energy and resources to provide for her baby. The body cannot afford the energy drain of menstruation or the demands of another pregnancy. So prolactin acts on the hypothalamus and the pituitary to inhibit the release of FSH and LH. This causes amenorrhea. As long as the baby continues to suckle, menses will not start. Ideally, periods should begin again when weaning is over, but often the timing is not that perfect.

In some women, high levels of prolactin will be present without pregnancy occurring. This will cause milk production and amenorrhea. If you notice a milky discharge from your breasts and have been amenorrheic for some time, it is possible that you are suffering from too much prolactin. Your breasts will seem firm and you may find that your clothes get damp from the breast discharge, although some women with this condition do not even notice the discharge. This condition is called *galactorrhea,* and it indicates a hormonal disorder. Why does this happen?

It is possible that small tumors called microadenomas are causing the increase in lactotroph cells. They are not really tumors but a small group of cells that reside in the pituitary gland. They are almost always harmless and can be treated. The tumors that are more dangerous are called macroadenomas. They are much larger than microadenomas, and if they are left untreated, they are likely to spread to other parts of the body. They can also press against the optic nerve, causing headaches and loss of vision. It is vital that medical treatment be sought if macroadenomas are suspected.

Some medications can also increase prolactin levels and cause hyperprolactinemic amenorrhea. Certain major tranquilizers, antidepressants, and blood pressure medications will suppress menstruation. If you are taking medication and are amenorrheaic, you should have your prolactin levels checked to see if the drugs are causing the disorder.

Stress, alcohol consumption, polyps in the mammary glands, and fibrocystic disease can also cause hyperprolactinemic amenorrhea. A clear sign is a milky discharge from your breast, although sometimes a woman may not notice it at all and still have high prolactin levels. Generally, treatment can be administered when advice is sought early enough. If you ever notice any kind of continuous discharge from your nipples, see a doctor at once. If this discharge is not milky but bloody, immediate treatment is vital because it could indicate a malignant growth.

Problems with the Thyroid Gland

Another cause of elevated prolactin is an underactive or malfunctioning thyroid gland. Some women have low levels of thyroid hormone circulating in their blood and it makes them feel unwell. If your thyroid gland is not producing enough thyroid hormone, the hypothalamus, detecting insufficient levels in the blood, sends a signal to the pituitary telling it to release thyroid stimulating hormone (TSH). TSH then tries to stimulate the thyroid gland to produce more thyroid hormone. The problem is that TSH also stimulates the pituitary to release more prolactin and prolactin levels shoot up preventing ovulation (see the description in the previous section).

If an underactive or an overactive thyroid gland is causing amenorrhea, you may experience weight gain, anovulation, puffiness, and fatigue. Hot flashes are also associated with this condition, as are bulging eyes, excessive sweating, nervousness, and decreased efficiency at work. Low energy levels can lead to a depressed immune system and vulnerability to illness and infection. Early diagnosis and treatment to restore the reproductive cycle are important.

Problems with the Hypothalamus

When the hypothalamus does not make enough of the brain hormone GnRH to stimulate the pituitary to make FSH and LH, ovulation cannot occur and we have the condition known as hypothalamic amenorrhea. Almost every one of us at some point in our menstruating years will experience hypothalamic amenorrhea from the very mild (when your period is a few weeks late), to the more severe (when it is a few years late).

When hypothalamic amenorrhea occurs, your cycle never starts at all. Even more mysterious than this malfunction is amenorrhea caused by a missing mid-cycle rise of LH. Lacking LH, the egg is never released from the follicle, and no progesterone is produced in the second half of the cycle. Depending on how high the levels of estrogen are in the blood, the endometrium will begin to develop, but the lining in the womb cannot be shed without medication.

The problem here seems to lie in the relationship between the ovary and the pituitary gland. There is a breakdown in communication between the two, and LH is not released in the middle of the cycle as it should be. Androgenic disorders could be causing the problem (see the next section). Stress and weight problems may also be contributory factors but there is no real evidence to support this. The problem remains a mystery.

Problems with the Adrenal and Ovarian Glands

"I spend my life looking in my hand mirror to check my facial hair," says Laura, who is twenty-nine and amenorrheaic. For the last four years she has been desperate to do something about the facial hair growth on her chin and cheeks. She has tried electrolysis for a year now, but the treatment is not effective and she still has to shave every day.

Laura's problem is not unusual although she thinks it is. Many of us suffer from facial hair growth, but because it seems so "unfeminine" we are very discreet about it. We make sure that through constant bleaching, plucking, and shaving the problem is never visible. We are also too embarrassed to discuss the hair growth, and so little attention is brought to our problem. The medical term for this is hirsutism. Hirsutism is also caused by serious hormonal disease such as a tumor in the ovary or pituitary gland.

Some of us may not suffer from hair growth but from outbreaks of acne that make us feel unattractive. Pimples, acne, and large red swollen bumps can develop on the skin, especially on the face, causing irritation and pain and possible scars when they have healed. Sometimes acne will also occur underneath the arms and in the groin area or underneath the breasts. There could be pus, swelling, and abscesses, and the infections may lead to fever and weakness. If you are lucky enough to escape serious bouts of acne and infection, you will still have a pale, dull complexion.

Others are concerned about thinning hair and fear eventual baldness. We may suffer from any or all of these problems as well as being amenorrheaic.

The reason Laura is amenorrheaic and suffering from embarrassing facial hair growth is that her body is being excessively affected by hormones called androgens, hormones that are produced by the ovaries and the adrenal gland. Their function is to stimulate hair follicles and sebaceous glands. Hair follicles grow hair, and sebaceous glands produce oil on the skin. For some reason, as yet unknown, the adrenal or ovarian glands will sometimes release a proportion of androgen hormone into the blood that is too high. One effect of elevated androgen in the blood is that the hormone hinders the release of the egg from the ovary. In a normal cycle it is believed that estrogen, followed by a spurt of LH into the blood, causes the egg to be released from its follicle. Androgen seems to hinder the estrogen spurt so that no LH is present to cause ovulation.

High blood pressure can be associated with adrenal hyperplasia and androgenic disorders. The elevated androgen may cause you to have a poor cholesterol profile and make the risk of heart disease high. Anovulation is usual.

Cancer of the lining of the womb is the greatest risk for women with androgenic disorders, since anovulation prevents the monthly shedding of the womb lining. Infertility is not usually the outcome, and treatment methods for androgenic disorders have a very high success rate.

What is the cause? Stress and disordered eating may again be the culprits here, although this is by no means a proven fact. It is likely, though, that after years of stress the adrenal gland just goes into overdrive and ovulation stops. The lack of ovulation causes the ovaries to secrete too much androgen and there is now androgen circulating from both ovaries and adrenal glands. Weight gain is possible because the androgen's affect on the metabolic rate makes appetite increase. Putting on weight makes the problem worse, but if you are very overweight in the first place you are also more likely to get polycystic ovary syndrome (PCO). Being obese causes insulin levels to be higher than normal, and insulin can stimulate the ovaries to produce more androgens.

Androgens are sometimes called "the male hormones," but all of us have them. They are responsible for the appearance of pubic hair and for the oiliness of the skin that occurs at puberty. If you have an endocrine disease your androgen levels may be as a high as those of a man, but this is very rare. Even if your levels are higher than normal for a woman, you still have far less androgen circulating than a man. Testosterone is the most powerful androgen and the most well known because it is what some weight lifters foolishly take to gain weight and build muscle. If a woman takes testosterone, she is likely to become amenorrheaic and may continue to have problems even after she stops.

Adrenal Gland Disorders

Androgens are produced in both the ovary and the adrenal gland. Levels of androgens rise at puberty and then plateau in the teens and fall naturally as menopause approaches. Androgenic problems in the adrenal and ovarian glands occur simultaneously, but problems specific to the adrenal glands are less likely to cause amenorrhea.

Adrenarche is the name given to the overproduction of androgens in the adrenal gland. In this case, at puberty the increase in androgen production is exaggerated in the adrenals and a disorder results. If the condition is very severe, amenorrhea occasionally occurs, although infrequent periods are more usual. Congenital adrenal hyperplasma is another cause of adrenal androgen excess. This is often detected at birth, and development of the genitalia is affected although it may also have a later onset. Adrenal hyerplasma will cause irregular periods and affect fertility. It is the result of an enzyme blockage that causes the overproduction of androgens.

Another problem with the adrenal gland that can cause amenorrhea is when the adrenal gland makes too much of its major hormone, cortisol. The sign of too much cortisol is weight gain, amenorrhea, and acne, so it may often be confused with the more common androgenic diseases. Most of us think of adrenaline rather than cortisol as the hormone that helps the body deal with stress and danger, but it is in fact a combination of both. Adrenaline helps you react instantly to the situation and decide to flee or fight, and cortisol gives you the strength to flee or fight. If a woman is constantly under stress the body will keep needing more and more cortisol, and this negatively affects ovulation.

Ovarian Androgen Disorder

When there is an ovarian androgen disorder the pituitary gland and ovaries do not interact normally. Polycystic ovary syndrome (PCO) is an extremely complicated disorder, but basically, the excess androgen from the adrenal glands and the ovaries is converted into estrogen. The brain, detecting the estrogen increase, suppresses FSH and increases LH, thus sending a confused signal to the ovaries. The follicles start to mature but never ripen, and without the LH surge, they are never released. The ovary begins to produce more androgen. Over time more and more underdeveloped follicles build up, giving the ovary a cystlike appearance. The outer lining of the ovary becomes thick and inhibits ovulation, making it hard for the eggs to break out. When follicles do not mature they remain in the ovaries and continue to make hormones. A woman who has PCO has follicles with an increased numbers of cells that make androgens.

Amenorrhea is usual when PCO is the case. Obesity, male hair growth, and endometrial cancer are all associated with the condition. It is also possible that the condition is inherited; research is being conducted to try to establish if this is indeed the case.

It is estimated that 5 to 10 percent of all women have some form of PCO. If this is so, then it is the most common cause of irregular periods and amenorrhea. The amenorrhea may not always be a long-term condition; you might find that you are amenorrheaic for several months and then get a very heavy, long period to be followed by months of amenorrhea again.

PCO often causes women great alarm and anxiety, partly because the word cyst makes us think of tumors. Cyst is really an unfortunate name for what is just an unusual appearance of the ovaries that can be treated effectively. Not all women with PCO have detectable cysts in their ovaries, and some women with cysts menstruate normally. Should tumors occur in the ovaries or adrenal glands, they will cause androgen excess. Tumors are what we all fear, but do remember that the condition is very rare. If you have too much male hormone you should not think that cancer is inevitable.

Premature Ovarian Failure

You are in your late twenties and your periods have stopped. You know you can't be pregnant. Would it perhaps occur to you that you might be in early menopause? This is exactly what happened to Sally.

> Sally's periods stopped when she was twenty-eight, but as she was involved in a lot of athletics and her life was busy, it didn't greatly concern her. It was when she started to have difficulty sleeping and was plagued with fatigue that she finally went to see a doctor. The doctor ran a series of tests, one of which included a check on her FSH and LH levels. They came out very high, and the doctor explained to her that they were high because they were trying to make her reproductive system work, a common symptom of menopause. He concluded that her lack of menses and lack of estrogen production meant that she was in menopause. Sally was devastated and is still in therapy to try to come to terms with what has happened to her.

Menopause usually occurs around the ages of forty-five to fifty-five, but for a small percentage of women it can happen earlier. There are even cases recorded of it happening to girls at the age of twelve. Because it seems unnatural, it is something many of us fear. Some 2 to 5 percent of women do go into natural menopause before the age of forty. All the signs of lack of estrogen occur (see Chapter 10). The ovary can't make its own hormones anymore and menstruation stops.

When premature ovarian failure occurs it can be terrifying. This is partly because of the negative associations our culture still has about women and aging. Menopause should not mean an end of productivity and sexuality as it still does to many. It is a perfectly natural phase in a woman's life, and just because child bearing is no longer possible it does not mean that we have nothing to contribute and can find no fulfillment; quite the reverse is true. But, if menopause is still hard for many of us to adjust to mentally and physically when we are in our forties and fifties, imagine how devastating it is when it happens ten or fifteen years earlier than it should!

Having your own natural child is no longer possible after menopause, but a full and happy life is still possible if you are given correct hormonal supplementation and lead a healthy lifestyle. You will not look any older. Menopause and aging are not the same thing. Women, like Sally, in earlier-than-normal menopause will show no signs of premature aging and will still look and behave the young age that they are.

There are several reasons why premature ovarian failure can occur. First, some forms of cancer treatment can bring on early menopause. Radiation treatment contains toxic substances that are harmful to growing cells and affect the ovaries. In other cases, an autoimmune disorder occurs and a woman's antibodies become confused and start to attack her own ovaries, adrenal glands, and thyroid gland, as if they were foreign and harmful presences. As a result, they can't function properly anymore. Savage syndrome or resistant ovary syndrome also causes premature ovarian failure. This is when the ovaries are filled with follicles that cannot mature. They cannot respond to FSH and LH and cannot release an egg. Why this happens is unknown. In other cases a woman may have a genetic disorder with an irregularity in her X chromosome. This is what happens in Turner's syndrome. Turner's syndrome is one of the most common of human genetic disorders and affects about one in four thousand girls in the United States. In Turner's syndrome one of the two X chromosomes is lost in early development, so the egg cells in the ovary, lacking the usual second X chromosome, dwindle rapidly until none are left. Finally, although there is yet no real medical proof, we do know that severe cases of eating disorders, stress, overexercise, and weight gain—all of which cause amenorrhea—are also associated with an increased likelihood of early menopause.

Early menopause and why it happens is a mystery of nature. In some cases it can be reversible, but it many others it is not.

Sometimes steps can be taken to prevent complete infertility, and you may still be able to have your own child from your own eggs. If correct treatment, self-care, and a positive approach are applied, early menopause should not be associated with aging or poor health.

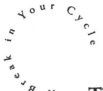
The Medical Effects of Amenorrhea

WHETHER YOU HAVE A PERIOD OR NOT IS LOGICALLY only significant if you are trying to get pregnant. Being amenorrheaic should not alter or limit how you feel in any way, and in some cases, like those of professional athletes, it may even lead to better physical performance. So, unless you wish to conceive, why concern yourself? It seems almost irrational to complain about the absence of a bodily function that we don't really need to sustain life and that can be inconvenient, uncomfortable, and painful.

Several decades ago this may have been the prevailing opinion among medical professionals, but nowadays, due to a developing understanding of how important a woman's menstrual cycle is to her health and well-being, doctors who dismiss the condition are rare. According to an interview with Dr. James W. Douglas, a much-respected reproductive endocrinologist and infertility specialist at the Plano Medical Center, Texas, "If amenorrhea has been present for more than six months she should see a doctor, even if she is not trying to get pregnant."

Regular menses are a good indicator of your general health and physical well-being. It is more natural and healthy for women to have their periods. Why? Because the menstrual cycle is regulated by hormones, and stable hormone levels are essential for good health. As Dr. Douglas notes, missed periods indicate some kind of hormonal malfunction and that "one of the bodily functions is not working right, because you are supposed to have a period every month. It's how the body was designed."

Hormonal Imbalance

Not all women with amenorrhea suffer from a hormonal imbalance, but many do. If you miss your periods regularly, or have been amenorrheaic for several months or longer, hormonal imbalance is likely. Somewhere, the hypothalamic-pituitary-ovarian axis has been disturbed and normal hormonal production suspended. As a result you become deficient in the important female hormones, estrogen and progesterone, which regulate the menstrual cycle.

Why are hormones so important? Hormones belong to the endocrine system, which—like the nervous system—directs and coordinates the systems of the body. The structures that make up the nervous system are visible, whereas as hormones are not. They are invisible messengers that go about their work in a mysterious, hidden manner, even though we can feel their effects every day in our lives. These effects should not be underestimated; they are dramatic and can be seen in our growth and development. In fact, hormones are so important that if you understand how they function, you understand how your body functions and why sometimes you feel the way you do. For women, the menstrual cycle is the most obvious way we feel the effects of hormones in our bodies, but for both sexes hormones are what make us what we are: a man or a woman.

Estrogen Deficiency

Estrogen is the hormone that feminizes the body. It gives you a female shape with breasts, hips, and buttocks, and it is in charge of the development of the reproductive organs, the thickening of mucous inside the vagina, and the growth of the womb lining.

If you suffer from severe hypothalamic amenorrhea that is stress related or from excessive levels of prolactin in your system, or if you are in early menopause, you will probably be deficient in estrogen to some degree. The effects of estrogen deficiency are sometimes not easy to detect, and some of you may still think, as many did in the past, that they are "all in the mind"; we now know that this is not the case. Depending on the length of your amenorrhea, and how estrogen-deficient you are, you might experience to a varying degree of severity some of the symptoms associated with estrogen deficiency—namely mood swings, hot flashes, a dry vagina, and generally feeling under the weather.

Do these symptoms sound familiar to you? If they do it is because estrogen deficiency symptoms are what we all experience at menopause. The risks of estrogen deficiency have now become common knowledge. Television commercials, advertising campaigns, and best-selling books are devoted to the subject in an attempt to increase awareness. For instance the Wyeth-Ayerst Women's Health Research Institute—for the discovery and development of medicines that help women lead healthier lives—produced in December 1997 an advertisement that was featured prominently in the weekly *TV Guide*, read by millions of Americans. The advertisement was striking. A faceless, naked female body with the brain, heart, and reproductive organs were highlighted, and arrows pointed to the sex organs, eyes, teeth, bone, and colon with a brief factual warning about how estrogen deficiency affects these vital organs. The message is to "Talk to your doctor" because problems with estrogen deficiency affect the entire body.

Most of the publicity about estrogen deficiency is targeted at women going through menopause, but if you have been missing periods for some time it is likely that you too will experience some of the symptoms associated with menopause, even though you may not be in menopause.

THE SYMPTOMS OF ESTROGEN DEFICIENCY You may find that your cup size decreases and that you lose weight around the hips and buttocks. Your initial delight over the weight loss is counterbalanced by the fact that you feel less feminine. Ongoing research also continues to investigate problems with vision and tooth loss in estrogen-deficient women. There may be a change in your skin texture, too. It looks dry and feels less flexible. Perhaps your hair loses some of its rich texture and starts thinning out as well. With all these subtle bodily changes taking place, you could start looking a little older than you are.

Many estrogen-deficient women also complain of vaginal dryness and thinning, which can be very uncomfortable. Vaginal mucus has an outer layer of cells that are sensitive to estrogen and decline when it is absent or deficient. Estrogen deficiency does not decrease sex drive but it will affect how moist the vagina is. Without estrogen the vaginal wall is thin and dry, making intercourse less enjoyable and lubricants necessary.

Another consequence of vaginal thinning is a thinning of the urethral tissues. You will need to pass urine more frequently. Estrogen loss can also increase the frequency of vaginal infections, which could also interfere with intimacy. In addition, the risk of colon cancer seems to be higher when you are estrogen deficient.

In the last ten years research has also explored questions surrounding the consequences of estrogen loss and cognitive functioning, memory, and Alzheimer's disease. You may find that you start forgetting things. You go to the shopping mall only to forget the reason you went there in the first place. Dates and names become vague, and you even find tasks like paying your bills on time, remembering where you parked your car, or planning your weekly schedule problematic.

Another unfortunate effect of estrogen deficiency is that the tissues of our bodies require estrogen to be healthy. From adolescence, our bodies need estrogen. If levels are too low you will feel unwell, and if levels are too high there are also problems such as nausea and breast tenderness. Only when estrogen levels are stable do we feel really well. If you are amenorrheaic you may feel less healthy and energetic than usual.

Some of the most common symptoms of estrogen deficiency are hot flashes, chills, and sweating— usually involving the head and neck. They may often occur at night, causing you to throw off your covers and sweaty sheets, only to find that you feel very chilly after a few minutes. Without estrogen, the body seems to operate at a lower heat level, and you may find that places you once felt comfortable in now seem stuffy and hot. When you have a hot sweat, the body is trying to rid itself of excess heat by making the heart beat faster so that more blood comes near the skin's surface. Sometimes the process is too efficient and you feel chilly soon after.

THE HIDDEN DANGERS OF ESTROGEN DEFICIENCY

Dr. Douglas says: "Most women don't necessarily show outward signs of estrogen deficiency. Women who experience outward signs of estrogen deficiency are those that have previously had high levels of estrogen. A woman who has primary amenorrhea, or who only menstruated for a brief time before amenorrhea set in, may never have had high levels of estrogen in the first place so her body won't know the difference. She will still be at risk of heart disease and bone .

loss, though. By far the biggest two health risks of hypothalamic amenorrhea are osteoporosis and heart disease."

Perhaps you don't actually feel unwell or notice any physical symptoms associated with severe estrogen deficiency, but you are still putting your health at risk. Amenorrheaic women are far more likely than women with normal menstrual function to develop the two diseases that kill millions of women every year: heart disease and osteoporosis.

INCREASED RISK OF HEART DISEASE Estrogen deficiency in women and heart disease are thought to be linked. Women in menopause who go on estrogen-related therapy are believed to have less risk of heart disease than those who do not.

Why is estrogen such a preventive measure? Because it is believed that in the absence of estrogen, which enables the arteries to carry more blood, constriction of the arteries can occur, causing heart attacks.

Estrogen deficiency is also thought to cause an increase in cholesterol levels. Without the protective effect of estrogen, cholesterol will damage the walls of the arteries and cause blockage. Cholesterol is impossible to avoid totally because it is made in the body, although you can cut down how much you ingest in food. Animal fat is the main source of dietary cholesterol—eggs, cheese, dairy products, and meat such as beef and pork. Our bodies need cholesterol to make hormones. It is only harmful when levels are too high.

More women than men die from heart attacks every year, and heart disease is the number one killer of women. Estrogen deficiency is not the only cause of heart disease; other factors such as environment, age, ethnic background, high blood pressure, body weight, diabetes, diet, alcohol, cigarettes, lifestyle, and family history also need to be considered as potential risk factors.

Heart disease kills five times as many women as breast cancer, about one in ten women. This is an alarmingly high number. All women should be educated about cardiovascular health. Estrogen seems to offer a protective effect against the disease, and any woman who is amenorrheaic should make sure her estrogen levels are assessed.

Regular menstrual function—as well as a balanced, healthy lifestyle and diet with moderate exercise levels—is the best way to ensure against heart disease. If you are amenorrheaic, perhaps the greatest danger you face is the possibility of heart disease. It is important to see a doctor and have your estrogen levels checked.

INCREASED RISK OF OSTEOPOROSIS

Lucy is twenty-one. She was amenorrheaic for twelve years because of an eating disorder. She suffers from chronic lower back pain. Her major concern is no longer dieting, but simply getting through the day with as little pain as possible.

Mandy is twenty-six and a competitive marathon runner who is amenorrheaic every training season. Ten months ago she broke her foot and has not been able to run since.

Sophie was thirty-five when she broke three ribs falling down in a shopping mall. She has a history of amenorrhea that dates back to her early teens.

These young women suffer from osteoporosis because they have been amenorrheaic. But isn't osteoporosis supposed to happen to old ladies?

We all know the "poor old lady" who is so stooped that she has to walk with a cane, her eyes lowered to the floor. She always walks very slowly, and it is obvious that sometimes she feels pain. "Isn't getting old sad?" we think to ourselves, taking it as a given that when we get older we too will become "little old ladies."

The idea that frailty and weak bones are part of the natural aging process has contributed to the trivialization and neglect of osteoporosis. Osteoporosis is not inevitable. Medical research has uncovered the causes of osteoporosis, can determine which of us are at greater risk of developing it, and has proven that it is a preventable disease. We don't all need to become frail old ladies who limp through our days in pain. We can prevent this from happening to us if we just gain greater understanding of what causes the condition and what we can do to prevent it from happening to us.

Osteoporosis is a disease in which low bone mass and a deterioration of bone tissue lead to bone fragility and a consequent increase in the risk of bone fractures. You could call it a disease that affects bone formation and structure and consequently the entire skeleton. Bone strength decreases and the skeletal framework supporting your body begins to deteriorate and become weak. Fractures and broken bones are very likely. These are often not even due to injuries or accidents, when the bones receive a forceful blow, but to simple everyday tasks such as bending or reaching. The bone loss of osteoporosis affects the whole body, and fractures are most common in the bones that support our structure: the spine and the hip. Wrist fractures are also quite common since the wrists can take the greatest impact from a fall. They are not as lethal as spine and hip injuries can be, but they are still extremely painful.

Spinal fractures typically occur without any blow or injury when a bone, or vertebra, in the spine gets so weakened by the decay that it will break during everyday activities like getting dressed or doing housework. Pain from spinal fractures is excruciating, and a woman can only heal with bed rest, which may take up to six months or longer. Even when healed, the woman will still find sitting painful and lingering discomfort will probably remain. Every time a vertebra breaks in the back there will be a loss of height, because the spinal curve changes, causing pain in the front of the chest, a protruding stomach, the loss of a waistline, and a head thrust forward. This abnormal posture can also cause problems with the head and neck.

Hip fractures result chiefly from falls. The bone that in fact breaks is the femur, the large bone in the thigh. Tragically, hip fractures often leave the individual permanently handicapped and unable to walk without a cane. Other complications, like blood clots, can develop as a result of the fracture. More often than not women die from complications as a result of the fall than from the fall itself.

The number of osteoporosis-related injuries and deaths is incredibly high. This is not really surprising considering that the disease affects more than twenty-five million people in the United States.

The process of developing a healthy skeleton begins before conception. Genetics play a role in the amount of bone density individuals will attain in their life. During growth and development, exercise and nutrition have an important part in bone formation, and peak bone mass is achieved by the age of thirty. After that a gradual decline will occur, and this becomes accelerated in females after menopause. Within bones there are living cells called osteoblasts, whose function it is to make or form new bone. Other cells called osteoclasts break down old bone. This process of formation and absorption takes place throughout our lives, but in the very young, more new bone is made than destroyed. The bone density of young adults is continually increasing until peak bone density is reached and more bone absorption occurs. Replacing old bone with new bone is necessary regardless of age as bones are affected by wear and tear and must be replaced. Osteoporosis occurs when there is an imbalance in the bone remodeling process. Too much bone absorption occurs, or too little bone formation occurs, and we have gradual bone loss.

Osteoporosis is a major cause of disability and death in women, killing more than breast cancer but not quite as many as heart disease. It causes pain, fear, and loss of independence.

Every woman is at risk for osteoporosis. Women who are Caucasian have a 54 percent chance of having an osteoporosis fracture—that is one out of every two women. One out of every three is expected to have a spinal fracture, and one out of every six a hip fracture. Some women who have these fractures can no longer care for themselves and must enter nursing homes.

Most of the thousands and thousands of individuals who die from osteoporosis every year are women. Why are we more at risk than men?

There is no one cause of osteoporosis, but some people are at greater risk of osteoporosis than others. Risk factors associated with the development of osteoporosis include race, age, calcium deficiency, diet, family history, alcohol, cigarettes, and lack of exercise—but being a female comes first. Eighty percent of sufferers are female, and because of this fact the disease has become known as a "woman's disease." The reason we are more prone to osteoporosis is because girls tend to build less bone than boys. We also become calcium deficient earlier than boys, and when we reach menopause our bone density loss increases again due to estrogen deficiency.

Statistics associated with osteoporosis in young women are not as well documented as those in post-menopausal women, but young women can lose up to 6 percent of their bone mass every year. Osteoporosis does not only happen to old women. If you are amenorrheic, your risk factor is high. You could be vulnerable to broken bones, curvature of the spine, and joint deformities.

How is osteoporosis connected to amenorrhea? If you are not menstruating you are likely to become estrogen-deficient. Without estrogen, the osteoclasts, the bone destroyers, seem to become more active than the osteoblasts, the bone creators. The imbalance causes the bones to weaken over the years. This is one of the reasons why at menopause, when we are estrogen-deficient and at risk of osteoporosis, estrogen-related therapy is recommended. Research indicates that most of the bone loss we have in our lives will be due to estrogen deficiency.

If you become amenorrheaic in your reproductive years you are stopping, or slowing, the development of bone mass, and you may never reach peak bone density. The implications of this for amenorrheaic women are frightening. You are decreasing bone density at an age when bone formation should be occurring. The adverse affects of this failure to develop skeletal strength may well be devastating. An athlete, for instance, who has been amenorrheaic for many years due to her training regimen could lose as much as 25 percent of her bone density.

For your own sake, if you are amenorrheaic do not ignore the problem. If you do, there may well come a time—perhaps sooner rather than later—when you resemble that "poor old lady" with joint disorders, fractures, pain, discomfort, and dependency. You don't have to let this happen to you.

Progesterone Deficiency

Amenorrhea also causes progesterone deficiency. Estrogen deficiency inevitably results in progesterone deficiency. If you are not ovulating you will not be producing progesterone, and the long-term medical risks here are heart disease and endometrial cancer from overstimulation of estrogen without progesterone.

A recent study at the Harvard School of Public Health and Center of Prevention of Cardiovascular Disease has possibly come up with a connection between progesterone deficiency and heart disease. The area still needs greater study, but researchers working with heart cells found that the hormone inhibited the growth of smooth muscle cells on blood vessel walls, which can contribute to clogged arteries, the precursors to heart attacks and strokes.

Endometrial cancer, another killer, is the greatest risk associated with progesterone deficiency. Progesterone is necessary to prepare the body for pregnancy. Its effects are often uncomfortable. The bloating, cramping, nausea, and pain of periods is the result of progesterone. But, despite the discomfort, progesterone has another beneficial effect: it prevents cancerous changes in the lining of the uterus that would otherwise come under the influence of estrogen.

General Poor Health

Oriental medicine techniques emphasize the importance of human energy flow. Energy can be depleted or supplemented by what we eat, where we live, how we think, how we feel, and how we eliminate waste. Chinese and Indian medicine believes that when this energy flow becomes blocked, distorted, or imbalanced in any way, the body will suffer with disease and the mind with anxiety. Acupuncture is based on the principle of channeling energy flow and trying to correct the imbalance. The Ayurvedic system and yoga techniques are concerned with seven chakras or energy points on the body and the connections between them. Chinese herbal medicine works on the same principle of balance and correction of energy flow in the body. For Chinese doctors, a woman's menstrual cycle—the frequency of menstruation, its color, and its texture,—is a vital indicator of the health and well-being of the woman. In Ayurveda, amenorrhea also would be taken very seriously because it indicates energy flow that is blocked, causing an imbalance in the body that will affect the health of the whole female. Until the imbalance is corrected the woman will not be healthy.

Western medicine is only recently beginning to learn from these ancient systems and incorporating some of their thinking and practices to improve treatment methods. The clinical effects of amenorrhea certainly do seem to support oriental and Indian concepts about the importance of balance and correct energy flow for a healthy body and mind. Amenorrhea is no longer regarded as something that should not cause concern. Slowly doctors are recognizing that a woman who is not menstruating, and who is not pregnant or menopausal, is not in a good state of general health, and that the dysfunction will not just affect her reproductive organs but her whole body and her emotional state as well.

Infertility

The short-term effect of amenorrhea is infertility. If you are not menstruating regularly it is very likely that you are not ovulating. If no egg is released from the ovary to meet your partner's sperm, conception is impossible.

The issue of fertility may not be at the top of your list of priorities. Perhaps you are an athlete dedicated to your sport, a young college student eager to experience life, a busy executive for an international company. You think that you have all the time in the world, and the notion of motherhood hovers somewhere vaguely in the distant future. At present this may be so, but there will come a time in your life when you will have to decide if you want to start a family. You may decide not to, but at least you will want the opportunity to decide for yourself. If you are amenorrheaic there is no choice. Your body has decided for you. An amenorrheaic woman who does not ovulate is infertile. Your fertility is sleeping. You cannot decide to get pregnant until your amenorrhea reverses itself. Sometimes this will happen, but in some cases it does not. Traumatic and expensive fertility treatments may be needed to reverse the amenorrhea. The unnaturalness of the whole infertility workshop can cause great distress. Amenorrhea robs you not only of your ability to conceive, but your ability to choose to conceive when you want to.

Concern about fertility for amenorrheaic women is often an unspoken fear and often what prompts them to see a doctor. When menses do not return naturally, although in most cases they do, ovulation-inducing medications will be needed. For the great majority of amenorrheaic women, being amenorrheaic does not make them infertile, but it might make conception harder to achieve.

Risk of Pregnancy

Having outlined infertility, it may seem strange to mention the risk of pregnancy. Many women who are amenorrheaic think they have a safe form of contraception. But hypothalamic amenorrhea can suddenly reverse itself. Why this happens is unknown. It may be due to a reduction in stress levels and a more balanced healthy life, but whatever the reason, ovulation does sometimes switch back on again. Since ovulation occurs before menstruation you have no way of knowing that it has occurred, and pregnancy is possible.

Will Periods Ever Return?

In most cases of both long- and short-term hypothalamic amenorrhea, menses will return. As Dr. Douglas notes: "Under extreme stress—say your parents both die in a car crash—your periods may stop for three months. Stress affects the way the hypothalamus releases hormones. That kind of situation is always short-term. It is a reactive situation. The brain reacts a certain way and when the stressor is gone, or has gotten used to the stress, it returns to normal."

The majority of women who are amenorrheaic start ovulating again when either stress diminishes, weight is stabilized, or exercise is reduced. If menses do not return by themselves, hypothalamic amenorrhea can often be treated with fertility drugs that act on the hypothalamus to restore menstruation. Generally menses return when the system gets this trigger, but sometimes they do not because the brain has simply become used to the way things were and cannot orchestrate the menstrual cycle on its own anymore. When this happens fertility treatments will be needed to induce menstruation.

In rare cases, when the hypothalamus stops telling the ovaries what to do, even medications and fertility treatments will not be able to turn the hypothalamic function back on. According to Dr. Douglas, "There is concern about this, and the situation makes no logical sense." This usually occurs in cases of secondary amenorrhea when weight loss has been drastic and activity levels very high. Even if training stops and weight is gained, the hypothalamus just does not switch back on again. When the hypothalamus cannot be stimulated by medication to induce ovulation, injections and treatments will be needed to stimulate the pituitary gland. If a malignant tumor is present though, or you are in early menopause, the condition is not usually reversible.

As far as post-pill amenorrhea is concerned, periods almost always return. Dr. Douglas notes: "Some women go off the pill and they don't have a period. What happens is that the birth control pill tells the brain that there is plenty of estrogen, so the brain decides that it doesn't need to do anything. It basically turns off and gets used to that. So when some women stop taking the pill the brain just doesn't turn back on again. The pill is not to blame. Most women who had irregular periods before the pill will have had them

A Break in Your Cycle

after so we cannot blame the pill. In time, unless there is some serious disease or premature menopause, the brains of these women with post pill amenorrhea will turn back on again, perhaps with the help of medication and they will have periods again."

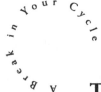

chapter 11

The Emotional Effects of Amenorrhea

THE HYPOTHALAMUS IS INFLUENCED BY ANXIETY AND unresolved conflict and pain, and menstruation can cease altogether for reasons that are linked to emotional stress. Polycystic ovary syndrome is also associated with alterations in brain chemistry. This strong connection between the menstruation cycle and a woman's emotional life is recognized in medical circles, but while numerous accounts are available of the bodily changes that occur with menstrual dysfunction, there are few about what actually goes on in the mind. How does being amenorrheaic make you feel?

The reproductive cycle involves far more than just the monthly shedding of blood for a woman during her reproductive years. Menstruation has an important biological function, but it is also a significant expression of maturity and sexual development. Growing into a woman involves menstruation, so it becomes part of what it means to be a woman. Understood this way, how you come to terms with your menstrual cycle—how you deal with it and feel about it—reveals much about what you think about yourself as a woman, how you feel about yourself now, how you feel about your past, and what attitudes, thoughts, and feelings will shape your future.

What does it mean to be a woman? This is one of the most complex questions you will ever ask yourself—one for which there will never be any one answer. Each woman will have her own answer, and just as our opinions and feelings constantly change, so too will the meaning we attach to our menstrual cycle at different stages in our lives. The only constant is that how you feel about menstruation right now relates to how you feel about yourself right now.

Reactions to Amenorrhea

Our feelings toward our menstrual cycle are unique and constantly changing, but it is possible to recognize certain emotional responses or tendencies in amenorrheaic women. The following responses are generalized for clarity, but they should give you some idea of the most likely reactions.

Concern

Your first worry is that you might be pregnant. This puts you in a stressful situation if the pregnancy is unwanted, or it raises false expectations. When you discover the truth you may feel either relief or sadness, but then concern again. Why doesn't your period come? Is some terrible illness or tumor infesting your body? You are not bleeding, so you know something is not right.

> "I felt bloated and edgy," says Sarah, who is twenty-nine and was amenorrheaic for two years. "If I wasn't bleeding every month I wondered where all the blood was going. I really thought that perhaps all the blood and toxins were collecting somewhere. I was really scared."

The belief that if a period does not start it must be lingering in the womb, or going elsewhere, is a common concern. It is an unfounded one though, because in most cases, unless something is obstructing the vagina, menstrual fluid is not retained. Generally, amenorrheaic women do not form menstrual fluid in the first place. The failure to release menstrual blood at the appropriate time can, however, cause tension and the false idea that somehow your system is blocked, because we have become programmed to expect a monthly bleed. In some cases hormonal imbalance does actually cause physical discomfort to some women (especially those with anovulation where the cycle tries to begin), but most amenorrheaics, for whom the cycle never starts at all, are less likely to experience physical symptoms because hormonal levels remain more static.

If you feel uncomfortable with missed periods it is because you know, even without referring to medical manuals for proof, that not menstruating is unhealthy. Menstruation is supposed to happen to women every month, and if you don't have your period you feel unnatural. Your response is a healthy, normal one. Don't think you are being paranoid. If you have not had a period for several months, your instinct to check things out as soon as possible with a doctor is right.

Another concern is early menopause. Have you been robbed of your right to bear children at such an early age? For most of us the monthly period is reassurance that we are healthy and have the potential for fertility. Being without it can cause great anxiety if you intend to start a family either now or in the future. The best thing you can do is stop worrying and see a doctor, who will find out the cause of your menstrual dysfunction and put your mind at rest.

Lack of Concern

Some women are not greatly concerned by absent menses. We are sure that in time nature will balance things out. We don't want to have a baby soon, and there is no major blood loss or feeling of ill health, so why worry? Maybe occasionally we experience mild concern, but not being sure if there is anything to worry about, we put off seeing a doctor.

This kind of response is both positive and negative. It's positive because often worry can make you feel worse, but it's negative in that you may be failing to seek treatment when treatment is necessary. Paying too much attention to variations in your menstrual cycle is not always helpful, but neither is paying too little.

Being so unconcerned about a bodily function that is dysfunctional may also indicate that you have a similar casual attitude toward other aspects of your life. Do you lack a sense of responsibility there too? Or are you one of those women who are always too busy with other things or constantly putting the needs of others before your own? If any of these are the case, a change in attitudes and a reassessment of priorities is important. Remember, nothing is ever as important as your own health.

Embarrassment

One woman expressed this common reaction: "When I first went to the doctor I felt embarrassed, not only because I wasn't normal and had no periods, but also because I had to talk about periods in the first place." There are still many of us who remain deeply embarrassed about a bodily function that is perfectly natural and totally feminine. Such attitudes are unhealthy and obsessive. All of us at some point in our lives have been embarrassed about having a period, especially when we were very young. The need for being discreet about bodily functions is part of being civilized, but a woman who feels embarrassed about menstruation is basically saying she feels embarrassed about being a woman. All of us should try to be a little more open and honest about a function that has allowed us to exist in the first place. After all, it is at the basis of all human life. It ensures the propagation of the species!

Relief

Michelle is stuck in a loveless marriage, feeling unfulfilled. She has big plans to leave her husband and get a job, but always finds excuses why she should not. She has been amenorrheaic for the past year.

Sandy has worked for years in the same tedious job. She blames her amenorrhea on the long hours she works. She knows that promotions should come her way but is fearful of asking for it or looking for a new job.

Kelly knows she should have left home years ago, but she doesn't know how she will cope in the world outside without the love and support of her family. Every Christmas she resolves to go to college next year, but she never gets around to making the arrangements.

Cara fears pregnancy and the burdens of motherhood and home. She presents herself for fertility treatment but has a terrible fear of putting on weight to make conception possible.

In the past, women did not have such a conscious struggle for identity as we do today. Life paths were planned out by parents, husbands, and society. A century ago we were not encouraged to think, express ourselves, work, make choices about our lives, be financially independent, or divorce. Things have changed now. At a very young age we are invited by society to go beyond the traditional role of being a woman. Our response to that invitation will be individual. A great many grasp the tremendous opportunities for self-development and challenge in the modern age, but some of us, perhaps influenced by years of conditioning about female stereotypes of helplessness and insecurity, lack enough confidence to do so.

If you are in a situation where you cannot make a decision, your

A Break in Your Cycle

body may stand still too and stop menstruating. You don't know what you want, you don't know how to be, you don't know what to do. The anxiety of indecision represses menstrual function. You feel relief from the confusing burden of womanhood and making decisions.

We all lack confidence to a certain degree, but unless we put ourselves in testing situations we will never develop. Change is an integral part of life; it's what makes the world go 'round. Often fear of failure, of making the wrong decision, prevents us from progressing and moving forward. But sometimes any decision is better than no decision at all.

Feeling in Control

Another unhealthy response to the female identity struggle is the obsessive desire for control. Maybe masculine ideals represent authority and control to you and femininity subordination and weakness. Without menstruation you feel you can aspire to masculine ideals, be more powerful, be in control.

You may think that you have power and control when you are amenorrheaic, but nothing could be further from the truth. Instead, you are living in limbo—a place where nothing can really happen because it is neither one thing nor the other. By suspending your female cycle you are really just putting your life on hold, living an existence that is disconnected and imbalanced. You will never find yourself by assuming a more masculine guise, and you will only come to terms with yourself when you accept fully who and what you are: a woman. And women menstruate. You may not like menstruation any more than you like death or illness, but it is a part of life. If you continue to resent your menstrual cycle, and what you perceive to be the limitations of womanhood, you are resenting and hating a part of yourself.

Whatever the reaction to being amenorrheaic, coming to terms with our sexuality and the menstrual cycle is a huge part of coming to terms with ourselves. Self-knowledge and creativity come only when we learn to respect our feminine rhythms and value being a woman. If you are missing periods, take a careful look at your attitudes. How do you feel about being a woman? How do you feel about yourself?

The Effects of Hormones

Karen, amenorrheaic for nearly two years, was bright, energetic, and outgoing and worked long hours for her demanding job in a publishing house. She began to notice that her
energy levels were not as high as they used to be. She had to
cut back on her activities outside work so that she could meet
the deadlines so often required of her. A Girl Scout leader in
the evenings, she found herself becoming increasingly snappy
and moody with the children. On the weekends all she wanted
to do was sleep because she was so exhausted. She longed to be
in a relationship but never seemed to meet the right man or
have the time to socialize and date.

Is Karen suffering from overwork, the demands of her busy sin-
gle lifestyle, or mild depression? Some would say that it is a combination of the three; others would say that there is some physical
reason for her low energy levels and fluctuating mood. Karen's fatigue, like eating disorders and depression, falls into that category
where medical opinion is still divided. How much of it is in the
mind, in the body, or a mixture of both?

The answer remains a mystery, but it probably lies somewhere in
between, since the mind and body are so firmly linked. Being amenorrheaic may not necessarily cause depression, but the unnatural
state of the body often indicates a hormonal imbalance, where estrogen is low and the risk of depression higher. Hormones affect
how we feel, think, and live. Our mood, energy levels, and lifestyle
will all be altered to some degree if hormonally there is an imbalance. Most amenorrheaic woman have some kind of hormonal imbalance.

How can estrogen deficiency influence mood? Hormones can affect how we feel and cause mood to be low. A low mood can lead to
decreased energy and possibly even depression. Research has proved
that depression can be caused by the depletion of certain chemicals
in the brain and that when these are readjusted mood improves.

Female hormonal levels will influence mood. Estrogen and progesterone have the ability to bind in the brain and influence brain
function. Estrogen can even alter the structure of certain brain cells
to make interaction with others easier, and it does affect brain sensitivity. Progesterone also acts on the brain but in a less decisive
manner. We do not know exactly how these hormones influence

mood but we do know that, just as they cause nausea and nipple enlargement, they also cause mood changes. Sometimes the physical symptoms of estrogen deficiency can affect mood. For instance, vaginal thinning may make sex less enjoyable, which may then lead to a loss of interest in sex and a decline in libido.

How your brain responds to estrogen and progesterone will influence your mood. For each woman the response will be different, from those who suffer the symptoms of premenstrual syndrome—including tears, fuzzy thinking, and depression—to those who have no discomfort at all.

Can we blame hormones then for feeling low? No, unfortunately we cannot. They play a part but not the major one. Why? Because hormonal changes will bring to our attention emotions that we have regardless of menstruation—including emotions that we have been repressing or ignoring. Your hormones make you more receptive and sensitive to what is there already. They heighten emotions and bring to focus aspects of our lives, or feelings we have, that are already causing frustration for us.

Being amenorrheaic places your body in an unnatural state and affects brain chemistry because of the hormonal imbalance. Your mood may become low as a result. If you have repressed emotions and feelings that cause pain and frustration, these are more likely to come to the surface and result in mood shifts and maybe even depression.

If your mood is low it will affect your whole lifestyle. Low mood equals low energy levels and fatigue, affecting how you eat and how you live. An unhealthy lifestyle makes you more vulnerable to infection and disease because your immune system is depressed.

Sexuality and Relationships

"I never felt really feminine," says Andrea. "All those years I was amenorrheaic sex became a little mechanical, really. I knew my partner liked it so that was enough for me. I got my thrills from pleasing, not from being pleased. I used sex as a way to feel close, for companionship, for human contact. When I finally got my periods back things changed. I still feel that sex is about intimacy, love, and giving, but I now find that I want to have some pleasure too."

Many women do report feeling less sexual when they are not menstruating. Although ovulation represents a peak in sexuality, women who menstruate can feel sexy at any point in their cycles. Amenorrheic women, however, without any cyclic changes, may find themselves losing interest in sex like Andrea did. This may be psychological because you feel less feminine without the potential for fertility, or it could be due to the absence of normal cyclic changes. The body is practical. Why send out signals for sexual arousal if pregnancy is not an option?

It is mistaken to conclude that if a woman rejects menstruation and cultivates a more androgynous body image she may have lesbian tendencies. This might be the case in rare instances, but many lesbians are very comfortable with their femininity and celebrate it. There is no proven link between amenorrhea and a tendency toward lesbianism. There are amenorrheic lesbians just as there are amenorrheic heterosexuals.

A woman who has been amenorrheic for some time may often feel incredibly lonely. Relationships, sexual and nonsexual, with both sexes become a problem. You don't have periods like other women anymore, so the empathy so important in female relationships is lacking, and you don't feel like a "real" woman as far as men are concerned. The result is isolation and loneliness.

Eating Disorders

"I was terrified of getting my periods back," says Rachel, who was anorexic from the age of sixteen to twenty-two. "If they ever came back it would mean the ultimate in failure. I thought about periods as a part of my old life as a fat person with no control or discipline. Without periods I was reborn clean, pure, and in control."

Amenorrhea is one of the symptoms of an eating disorder like anorexia and bulimia. Body weight falls too low for menstruation to occur, or the state of malnourishment the eating disorder has placed the body in is so severe that menses cease. Eating disorders have their basis in psychological problems.

The need to feel cleansed from basic bodily functions is part of the anorexic's struggle for freedom from the flesh. Flesh in their minds is base, nasty, uncontrollable—something to be conquered or escaped from. For bulimics, vomiting makes them feel a similar kind of relief that all the food has gone.   .

> "I would gag and gag and gag after my binges," says Linda. "I
> just had to feel that every bit of what I had taken into my body
> had been expelled. For a brief moment after I had finished I
> felt truly clean and pure again."

Victims of eating disorders are struggling for a sense of self.
The arena that they choose to find themselves in is not society or
relationships but food and body image. The loss of menses does not
greatly concern them; they are obsessed with food and the complicated emotions that it allows them to suppress and deny. The
problem with placing such an importance on food, though, is the
connection food has with nurturing, normality, and sharing. Food
will always bring to the surface the emotions they are trying to
escape from.

Eating disorders can have dangerous effects because of their psychological basis. Healing the body is never enough. You have to heal
the mind too, particularly the underlying issue causing such behavior. Usually, unresolved relationships with parents tend to be at the
bottom of the problem. Perhaps the victim's parents never had fulfilling lives and there is fear of surpassing them. Mother-daughter
relationships can be especially complex, and an anorexic can often
take on the burdens of her mother's life, identifying and sharing her
mother's hidden resentments and anguish. This is dangerous, unhealthy, and dysfunctional. The relationship will not get better but
worse by the daughter's attempt to extend her childhood so her parents stay together, feel needed, or feel that they are still young. In
other cases, tensions and problems within the family are kept hidden and unexpressed: a father who is too controlling, a mother who
is too manipulative, sibling rivalry. Whatever the reason, the victim
finds herself unable to live her life until the emotional issues trou-
bling her and those close to her are resolved.

Amenorrheaics who have severe eating disorders are in a dangerous state mentally and physically. Eating disorders lead to depression, lethargy, low self-esteem, weakness, high blood pressure, hair
loss, gall bladder disease, gall stones, heart disease, ulcers, constipation, anemia, dry skin, skin rashes, dizziness, reduced sex drive,
amenorrhea, gout, infertility, kidney stones, numbness in the legs,
compulsive eating, reduced resistance to infection, electrolyte

imbalance, bone loss, osteoporosis, and death. For whatever psychological reason the disorder has set in; unless emotional help and guidance is given not only will the victim of the eating disorder tear her life apart, but the lives of those around her, too.

The Emotional Effects of Pituitary, Thyroid, and Androgenic Disorders
Pituitary Disorders

As I have outlined previously, the discharge that comes from your breasts and the breast tenderness you feel may cause you embarrassment. The terrible fear of breast cancer will also be a source of great anxiety to you. You are probably also suffering from estrogen deficiency so you may experience some of the emotional effects of hormonal imbalance.

Thyroid Disorders

If you have an underactive or overactive thyroid gland, it is probable that you will feel sluggish due to weight gain. You may also be experiencing extreme fatigue. Debate still rages about whether chronic fatigue is a mental or a physical problem. There is no real answer to give here. If you have problems with your thyroid, treatment will help you with your energy levels, but it is also worth looking into other areas of your life, such as your work or your relationships, to see if perhaps they are contributing to your exhaustion.

Androgenic Disorders

Women with androgenic disorders may experience fertility problems, excessive hair growth, acne, weight gain, and hair loss, and they may have an increased risk of cancer in the womb. It can be a devastating disease. The physical symptoms of polycystic ovaries are well documented in medical textbooks, but less attention has been paid to the emotional effects of these symptoms. Infertility can occur with long-term polycystic ovaries, but the emphasis on fertility and the thousands of women who have conceived has shifted emphasis away from the other symptoms. Androgen disorders do not tend to affect a woman's sexuality and sex life, but the presence of body hair and acne could cause inhibitions.

Excessive hair growth on the face, back, or arms can be acutely embarrassing for women. Society regards hair as attractive on the face and chest of males, but on females hair is only considered attractive on the head and nowhere else. Millions of dollars are spent each year on hair removal cream and treatments for female body hair. Women shave their legs, wax their bikini lines, pluck their eyebrows, and keep a careful watch on any unsightly hair that is not where it should be. For women without androgenic disorders, shaving legs and underarms is a daily routine. For women with the condition, hair may start growing around the lips and on the side of the face, as well as elsewhere on the body. Feeling constantly ashamed of budding beards and mustaches, these women will spend hours each day shaving, plucking, and bleaching. Usually, the job is done so well that nobody notices the problem; this is perhaps the reason why the problem receives so little attention. Women who have male hair growth would rather nobody knew about it.

The emotional effects of excessive hair growth are not well documented, but one thing is clear: there will be suffering. Our society is not tolerant of women who deviate from the cultural idea of what is considered feminine. Female facial hair is such a taboo subject that women who have normal facial hair even worry that they might have a problem when they don't. Why? Because men are supposed to have facial hair and women aren't. Women in fact do get facial hair. It is normal to have some facial hair, but some of us get it in greater degrees than others, and women with androgenic disorders usually get it in excess.

Attitudes should relax a little about the stigma of female facial hair, because if you think about it our sharply defined idea of feminine and masculine is not as absolute as we like to think. Think of those men who have long, almost feminine hairstyles! If we continue to stigmatize and ignore the problem of facial hair we cause even greater pain and humiliation to women who are suffering enough already, through no fault of their own. More information and support should be made available for sufferers.

Although not quite as embarrassing as facial hair, acne can also cause women with polycystic ovary syndrome a great deal of discomfort, pain, and embarrassment. In severe cases depression and isolation can occur. People will not automatically think that there is a hormonal imbalance but may stare at or shun the sufferer, believing that a terrible diet or disease must be to blame.

Socially accepted ideas of feminine beauty not only stigmatize acne and facial hair, causing great pain to those who have it through no fault of their own, but a woman going bald is off limits too. Women of all ages worry about their hair—how much or how little they have—and it has great significance for feelings of well-being. If you are going bald or have very thinning hair, you may feel guilty that this frightens you more than other traumatic events in your life, like the loss of a loved one. You feel miserable, wretched, and extremely helpless, prepared to do anything to reverse the process. Treatments for hair loss are available, and usually the condition reverses itself, but in severe cases baldness can happen. The anxiety this causes will need sensitive handling and a careful reassessment of ideas about traditional female beauty.

The Emotional Effects of Post-Pill Amenorrhea

Sally feels like she is on an emotional roller coaster. At last she is in a position to start a family and all those years worrying about unwanted pregnancy are over. She goes off the pill but her periods will not start. She read somewhere that this is normal, but she gets impatient and anxious. After six months she wonders if they will ever come back, so she goes to a doctor, who tells her to wait a little longer. Every day she waits for a hopeful sign that her menses will return. She hears about women who are on the pill who got pregnant. She discovers that her best friend got pregnant the week after she stopped taking it. What is wrong with her? Sally goes back to the doctor, who advises tests and fertility treatment. She feels wretched. She never thought that she might be infertile. What did she do wrong? She thinks back to the years when she had a normal period and remembers how sick she was when she took her first pack of pills. She concludes that the pill must be to blame. The pill stopped her from menstruating. She gets angry and resentful and wants to know why the doctor who put her on the pill did not warn her that this could happen. What if her periods never come back?

Most women will resume normal menstrual function after coming off the pill, but a small percentage do not. As I have outlined earlier, the pill is not to blame for menstrual irregularities that occur when you come off the pill. All that it does is hide imbalances or problems that would have been there anyway. In most cases, menses will return with the correct stimulation from medicine. This may be so, but emotionally it is hard for some women to understand that after taking the pill their once-normal periods have disappeared. Anger, regret, resentment, confusion, guilt, and prejudice about oral contraceptives may follow.

The Emotional Effects of Irreversible Amenorrhea

Women should not be judged by the use they make of their reproductive organs. Centuries of conditioning have bound us to the idea that a woman's function is to reproduce, so it is never easy to come to terms with infertility. However, a woman who is childless can still adopt a child if she wishes, enjoy sexual and non-sexual relationships, and lead a rounded, satisfying life.

If you find fulfillment in your life, you are a living example that women who cannot be biological mothers have much to offer the world. Women who are "childless" give birth in other ways and liberate us fully from restrictive, traditional ideas about what it means to be a woman.

Early Menopause

"Everywhere I went," says Wendy, who went through menopause at the age of twenty-seven, "I saw women with babies. Even filling out forms that asked if I had any children caused me pain. I was too embarrassed to tell friends I was going through menopause, and for many years could not tell my Mom until her insistent "when you have children of your own" just got to me. She was even more devastated when I told her than I was, and the two of us cried for days. Something could never be born, but we acted as if someone had died. My boyfriend wanted children, so that relationship ended. Now, if I get into another relationship, I don't know when is the best time to talk about it. Sometimes I look into the mirror and see this old lady looking back at me. Nobody really understand how it feels to be in menopause when you are in your twenties."

There is always so much emphasis on women who conceive with the wonders of new fertility treatments—women who beat the odds—that the ones who don't are often ignored. It is believed that nobody wants to read about women who for some reason or other can't conceive. This emphasis on the belief that medical science can make anything possible, makes it exceptionally hard for women with premature ovarian failure who know that they will never be fertile again. At a far younger age than is normal they have to go through the emotional and physical changes of menopause. Although they will not look any older, they may feel it.

Menopause with proper hormonal treatment does not mean aging or wrinkles. If you have premature ovarian failure you will probably look and feel fine physically, but mentally and emotionally it will be a different matter. You will have to come to terms in your own way with the fact that you have gone through menopause early and cannot bear children. This is a powerful and distressing thought and, try as you might to be positive, images of decay, being shriveled up before your time, and sterility flash through your mind.

In centuries past a barren woman would have been excluded and marginalized from society—the spinster aunt everybody felt sorry for. Thankfully this has all changed, and we no longer equate child-bearing and fertility with having a successful, happy life. Many women who are fertile choose not to have families because they decide to focus on other areas of their lives. Unfortunately, for women with early menopause the choice is out of their hands, and they will need special care, therapy, and treatment to come to terms with it and discover that a fulfilled, happy life is still possible.

Summary

The emotional responses to amenorrhea that this section has highlighted are generalized to indicate likely—but by no means every—emotional responses to the condition. Perhaps you don't relate to any of the categories, perhaps you recognize some of the emotions expressed, or perhaps you are a mix of conflicting responses. All of us are different, but whatever your unique response, this section has demonstrated that amenorrhea sooner or later will cause you emotional distress of some kind.

The way to avoid the emotional anxiety of amenorrhea is the same as the way to avoid the anxiety caused by the physical symptoms: seek out medical advice. Go to a doctor, ask for help, and take a careful look at your lifestyle with a view to making positive changes.

A Break in Your Cycle

The following chapters of this book will look at the various treatments and advice available from doctors, both conventional and alternative, and suggest ways you can help yourself.

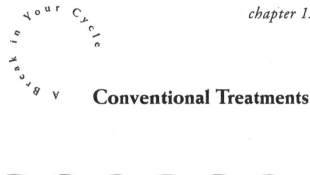

chapter 12

Conventional Treatments

IF YOU ARE AMENORRHEAIC YOUR RISK OF DEVELOPING heart disease, osteoporosis, and cancer significantly increases. Hormonal imbalance and the complications connected with it are also likely. In rare cases a serious disease or early menopause could be causing the menstrual dysfunction.

Perhaps you feel fine. There is probably nothing seriously wrong with you, but are you prepared to take that risk? Don't feel uncomfortable about seeking medical advice or think that you are wasting your doctor's time. Not having periods is a legitimate cause for concern, and your physician should take the matter seriously.

When to See a Doctor

If you are age sixteen or older and have never had a period, you are suffering from primary amenorrhea and should consult a doctor. Normal menstrual function should begin by or around age fourteen.

If you previously had periods but have stopped menstruating for the last three to six months, you are suffering from secondary amenorrhea and should consult your doctor.

If you are menstruating now but have a long history of amenorrhea in the past, you need to find out what your estrogen levels are so you can protect against osteoporosis and heart disease. You should also make sure you have regular Pap smear tests. A progesterone supplement may also be needed to keep the endometrium from overresponding and overgrowing, thus increasing the risk of cancer.

What to Expect

The first thing your doctor will want to know is whether you are pregnant or not. This will always be excluded first by physical exam and laboratory testing for pregnancy hormones. You probably know already that you are not pregnant, but your doctor will want to run checks to make absolutely sure.

Once it has been established that you are not pregnant, your doctor may tell you to come back in a few months and to watch your diet, exercise, and stress levels. If this is the case do not think that there is nothing to worry about. Until you get your regular periods there is cause for concern. Make absolutely sure that you keep your next appointment with your doctor.

When your amenorrhea has stretched over a six-month period, your doctor might continue to treat you or refer you to a specialist. The best person for an amenorrheaic to see is either a gynecologist, an infertility specialist, or a reproductive endocrinologist.

When you see your specialist or doctor, a thorough medical history will be required because amenorrhea is considered to be a symptom, not a cause. It is not a disease and it is not life threatening, but what causes it could be. Successful management of the problem depends on an accurate identification of the cause and an understanding of your individual needs. Amenorrhea may take some time to successfully diagnose. Treatment will not be administered until the cause is identified. To help your doctor identify the underlying causes, he or she will need to know all about your lifestyle and medical history. Various questions to expect will include:

- What is your menstrual history?
- How do you feel? Do you have hot flashes, decreased sex drive, weight loss or gain?
- Are you on any medication?
- Is your life stressful?
- How much do you exercise?
- What is your diet like?
- Do you smoke, drink, take drugs?
- Do you have any breast discomfort or milky discharge from your breasts?
- Do you have problems with facial hair, acne, hair loss?
- Do you feel tired all the time?

- Have you recently had any infection?
- Have you had any headaches or vision problems?
- Have you had surgery recently?
- What oral contraceptives have you been using?
- Is there any history of this kind of problem in your family?

What happens next will depend on the doctor. Every doctor will perform certain standard tests, but apart from the pregnancy test that always comes first, they may proceed in a different order from the one I describe in the following section. Amenorrhea is always a bit of a mystery. The doctor plays detective, searching for clues and eliminating all possible causes with tests for various conditions, until the culprit causing the problem is finally discovered and treatment can begin.

Diagnostic Approaches
Pregnancy Tests

Pregnancy must be ruled out before any treatment can be given. Some of the tests performed later may be harmful to a developing fetus. A physical examination can determine pregnancy because a soft cervix, full breasts, and an enlarged thyroid gland all indicate pregnancy, but a blood test and urine test will be more reliable.

Pelvic Exams and Pap Smears

The doctor will examine your reproductive organs to check for any abnormalities, cysts, or tumors that might be causing your amenorrhea. A Pap smear is necessary to check for cancerous cell growth that may occur when there is no monthly shedding of the lining in menstruation.

Thyroid Tests

An underactive thyroid gland can prevent ovulation by elevating prolactin levels and secreting insufficient thyroid hormone. When the thyroid is underperforming, the hypothalamus tells the pituitary to secrete more thyroid stimulating hormone. The problem is that the hypothalamus also gets the pituitary to stimulate more prolactin. High prolactin levels inhibit ovulation.

If this is your problem, the mystery of your amenorrhea has been solved. Thyroid disorders can be treated simply and easily with medication for the thyroid gland. Your metabolism and periods should return to normal with the medication.

Checking Prolactin Levels
Prolactin levels are checked to rule out hyperprolactinemia. Too much prolactin inhibits ovulation and often causes discharge to come from your nipples. A test will be run to measure the levels in your blood. If levels are elevated, this is the reason for the dysfunction. Sometimes a milky discharge from the breasts is present when there are normal prolactin levels. Why this happens is not clear, but it may be associated with stress, drugs, alcohol, high blood pressure, or an underactive thyroid gland. If the discharge from the breasts is bloody, a malignant tumor is present and will need urgent attention.

If you're fortunate, your breast discharge and elevated prolactin levels, if you have these symptoms, are due to harmless cell growths and not the more dangerous larger growths, which—if left untreated—can cause diabetes, headaches, vision loss, and life-threatening pituitary tumors. How the condition is treated depends on your age, medical history, tumor size, and the amount of prolactin in your blood. Therapies will include medication, surgery, or sometimes—if the growth is tiny—no treatment at all because the cell growths disappear on their own. Medication such as bromocriptine is usual. Bromocriptine imitates the action of dopamine, the inhibiting factor for prolactin in the pituitary, and lowers prolactin levels. The treatment is very effective, but it can cause side effects such as dizziness, headaches, and nausea. The side effects can be avoided by taking the medication via the vagina and by starting the treatment slowly.

Checking Medication, Diet and Substance Use
Some kinds of medication, frequently those for psychiatric treatment, prevent menstruation. Cigarettes, alcohol, drugs, and severe malnutrition can also have the same effect. If you are a heavy drinker or smoker, or use drugs this could be causing amenorrhea and you will be encouraged to lead a healthier lifestyle.

Body Weight

If you are seriously underweight your body fat levels are too low for menstruation, and if you are obese they are too high. If either of these are the case your doctor will recommend a sensible healthy weight gain or weight loss plan to restore menstrual function, but will also run other tests to see if any other complications have developed alongside the weight problem.

Recent Surgery

If you have had a dilation and curettage recently, or other types of uterine surgery, such as myomectomy or cesarean section, adhesions that might have formed (Asherman's Syndrome) should be checked out as possible causes of amenorrhea.

Going Off the Pill

If you have recently discontinued oral contraceptives and you have been amenorrheaic for less than six months, you may have to wait for future treatment. If it has been more than six months, the contraceptive you took is not related to your menstrual dysfunction and will be ruled out as a cause.

Treatments for Hormonal Imbalance

If the tests I've described come out negative and you do not demonstrate any obvious reason for amenorrhea, it is likely that hormonal imbalance due to hypothalamic, pituitary, or ovarian dysfunction is the problem.

Primary Amenorrhea

In cases of primary amenorrhea, the most common cause is hormonal imbalance. Your doctor will treat you with hormone therapy to stimulate sexual development and menstruation. Provided you have a healthy diet and lifestyle the treatment should be successful.

The Progesterone Challenge

If you have secondary amenorrhea and your doctor suspects hypothalamic dysfunction, the progesterone challenge test will be administered. In many cases this test will be one of the first tests you are given after the pregnancy test. You will be given a pack of pills that resemble oral contraceptives, and you will be told to take 10 milligrams a day for five or ten days. These pills, called Provera, are to test your body's response to progesterone. They may make you feel foggy, moody, and nauseous when you take them.

After finishing the medication you should bleed within two to five days. If there is any bleeding at all, the result is positive. Sometimes it may take an increased progesterone dose for this to occur. If after a sufficient progesterone challenge you do not bleed, the result is negative.

A POSITIVE RESPONSE If you bleed after the progesterone test you are not completely estrogen-deficient. The basic diagnosis at this point is anovulation, for which there are many causes. If there is a history of stress, weight loss, medication, drugs, or overexercise, this could be causing amenorrhea. Disorders such as polycystic ovaries, ovarian tumors, tuberculosis, thyroid disease, and diabetes should also be excluded.

TREATMENT OF POLYCYSTIC OVARY SYNDROME (PCO) If there is an excessive amount of androgen in your body, it will be converted into estrogen. Your brain, detecting the amount of estrogen, sends confusing signals to the ovaries, which cause them to malfunction. Follicles start to mature in your ovaries but fail to ripen, and without their release even more androgen is released. Over time the trapped follicles build up in the ovaries and cysts develop. These can often be detected by ultrasound, where the characteristic appearance of PCO is a ring of small to medium follicles around an enlarged ovary.

If you have PCO, it is likely that you have been suffering from excessive hair growth on the face and body, acne, and weight problems. As these symptoms can occur without PCO, your doctor will run a series of tests to see if the adrenal and ovarian glands are producing excess androgen or if tumors are present. If you have ovarian cysts your doctor will advise dietary changes and regular exercise as part of the treatment for PCO. Medication will also be needed to suppress adrenal androgen. In most cases medication is successful, but if it is not, surgery may be necessary. To combat the number of androgen-producing cells, fertility specialists may use laser treatment in the ovaries or resort to the old-fashioned method of surgically cutting a piece out of the ovaries.

Early diagnosis of PCO is vital to prevent permanent infertility and the terrible risk of cancer from the overgrowth of the endometrium. If androgen production is stopped early enough the ovaries will return to normal functioning and fertility will not be affected.

If PCO is not the case and you bleed after the progesterone challenge, it is possible that after this hormonal stimulation your reproductive system will start functioning normally again. If, however, periods do not return naturally, you will be put on hormonal therapy to correct the hormonal imbalance or be given fertility drugs. Fertility drugs, however, are only administered if you intend to get pregnant. Too much use of fertility drugs will make the ovaries resistant to them. Also the complications of amenorrhea—such as low estrogen levels and increased risk of heart disease—can be more directly dealt with by appropriate hormone treatment.

FERTILITY DRUGS If you want to get pregnant, the fertility drug clomiphene citrate can make many anovulatory women ovulate. Known as clomid, the drug stimulates ovulation in 75 percent of women who take it. It helps women whose ovaries make some estrogen but not enough to produce a sufficient estrogen surge to release FSH and LH.

How does it do that? We don't really know, but it is possible that because the drug competes with estrogen in the hypothalamus, it causes a release of FSH and LH from the pituitary when the course of clomid pills is completed. Follicles ripen as a result, and they release estrogen. The brain in response to the estrogen surge sends LH to the ovary, which triggers ovulation.

If you are to go on clomid your doctor will first give you Provera to make you bleed. Any day from the first to the fifth day of your bleed you will take clomid pills for several days. Ovulation usually occurs about seven days after you finish the clomid treatment. Your first dose of clomid will be 50 milligrams daily for five days. If you fail to ovulate and have a period, the dose will be increased to 100 milligrams. The maximum dose given is about 250 milligrams.

In some cases the egg ripens on clomid but you fail to ovulate. If pregnancy is desired, a shot of human chorionic gonadotrophin, the hormone that later indicates pregnancy, is needed. It comes from the urine of pregnant women and is similar to LH in that it can trigger ovulation. If clomid does not work for you, stronger fertility treatments will be needed.

Pergonal may now be used to stimulate ovulation, and it has a very high success rate. It is mainly used for women with low levels of FSH, LH, and estrogen. Pergonal will make your ovaries release several eggs because it contains human chorionic gonadotrophin, which supplies FSH and LH directly to the ovaries.

Fertility treatments are improving all the time, and a number of amazing drugs are available for women. Unpredictable side effects such as depression, pain from overstimulated ovaries, insomnia, nausea, hot flashes, and the risk of multiple births can occur with the medications. The symptoms are not usually serious, though, and if they make your periods come back or help you conceive, they are well worth taking.

A NEGATIVE RESPONSE If you do not bleed following the progesterone challenge, there is most likely a problem with your FSH level being either too high or too low. If your level of FSH is normal, then you may be given estrogen followed by progesterone to induce a period. If bleeding occurs, you have hypoestrogenism (a low estrogen status similar to menopause), and you will need estrogen-related therapy for your menses to return. If you still do not bleed, then obstructions like those caused by Asherman's syndrome need to be investigated. High levels of FSH will indicate that you may be in early menopause, which I will discuss later.

If your levels of FSH are low, you have severe hypothalamic pituitary failure. A pituitary tumor or chronic disease may be possible so levels should be checked, but more likely the failure is due to severe stress, dieting, strenuous exercise, or drugs.

Hypothalamic amenorrhea often has a stress-related cause. Even mild stress can inhibit menstrual function and affect your reproductive health. If the stress is very severe it can result in hypothalamic malfunction that can take a long time to reverse itself. In extreme cases it may never reverse at all, so that you become permanently amenorrheaic. To prevent the possibility of this occurring, early diagnosis of the problem is essential. Patients with eating disorders often have psychological problems, and they are often very hard for a doctor to treat. He or she will suggest lifestyle modifications and perhaps recommend a therapist or a psychiatrist.

Usually lifestyle changes, such as gaining weight or decreasing training intensity, will resolve your severe hypothalamic amenorrhea. If it does not, hormonal therapy will be recommended.

HORMONAL THERAPY This is necessary for women for severe hypothalamic amenorrhea, for those with irreversible amenorrhea, and for those who do bleed after the administration of progesterone but seem unable to have periods by themselves. Estrogen treatment will prevent the onset of bone loss, and reduce the risk of heart disease and cancer. You will be given estrogen and progesterone either by oral contraceptives, hormone therapy, or fertility drugs, unless a serious disorder is present that makes estrogen contraindicated, such as cardiovascular disease, diabetes, migraine, or epilepsy.

As well as reducing the risk of bone loss, and protecting against cancer and heart disease, oral contraceptives provide contraception. They will produce regular bleeding, but the dosage of estrogen and progesterone may need to be adjusted to make sure that a bleed occurs. Some side effects such as foggy thinking, nausea, and weight gain may result.

Birth control pills help the uterus shed its lining, but they also prevent ovulation. Because you have regular bleeds you may wrongly think that your body is being protected by the hormones. But if you continue to have disordered eating habits or train too hard, or if your stress levels remain too high, you are still harming your body and need to make a change.

If contraception and fertility are not the main concern, estrogen and progesterone therapy is given. This is the same treatment given to women who are in menopause because some amenorrheaics may have bone loss and estrogen-deficiency symptoms similar to menopausal women. Again the dose will have to be adjusted to the correct one for you.

Finally, if fertility is desired fertility drugs will be used (see page 127).

Treating Attitudes and Lifestyle

Is your diet so out of control (bulimia) or your body weight so low (anorexia) that you don't have periods anymore? Or are you so obese that food has become your only real pleasure in life?

Maybe you are an exercise addict who keeps on adding to your exercise routine so that it takes over your life. Worse still, are you both an exercise addict and a dieting fanatic?

You may not have a full-blown eating disorder like anorexia, but perhaps you belong to that group of women who have less severe but still destructive eating and exercise obsessions. You do eat, but your eating is disordered. You don't go to the extremes of a severe eating disorder victim, but you still dislike your body enough to punish it with dysfunctional eating and overtraining. You spend a lot of time obsessing about food. According to Francis Berg, editor of *Healthy Weight Journal,* people with eating disorders think about food 90 percent of the time, and dysfunctional eaters about 50 percent of the time. That is more than half your life spent obsessing about body image. You do not exercise or restrict your diet to feel healthy; you do it because you are terrified of gaining weight. In some cases the obsession gets so bad that feelings of well-being are based on how much has been eaten and how much exercise has been done. You often feel unwell, isolated, and depressed. Even worse, after a while you stop losing weight due to a slowed metabolic rate. This makes you panic, and now you really are vulnerable to developing full-blown eating disorders.

If you resist hormonal treatment because of the fear of gaining weight, therapy is needed because the desire to be thin is stronger than the desire for good health. Making changes in the body's hormonal balance is futile if unhealthy attitudes remain the same. Attitudes must change first, because often the mind-body connection in cases of hypothalamic amenorrhea is very strong. There is little respect or liking for the body, and such negative self-attitudes will influence brain and body chemistry.

For any treatment to be successful, the emotional problem causing the imbalance in your life must be treated also. If you have a severe eating disorder or an exercise addiction, you may be the hardest patient to treat because you have become inflexible and rigid in your regime. Food and body fat are the only areas in your life where you feel you have any control, so you resist attempts to change. A full recovery will depend on support from your family, friends, and doctor, but also on education about how to cultivate healthy attitudes. You need to start being kind to your body, eat sensibly, get moderate exercise and fresh air, reduce the stress in your life, and stop regarding body weight as the only standard for you to evaluate your self-esteem by. If you can't make these kinds of adjustments alone, therapy can help you understand why you dislike yourself to the point of pushing your body to dangerous extremes.

Counseling

You need to understand why you place such value on controlling your body. Perhaps you know why, but more often than not you don't. You were not abused as a child or raped. What is causing you to behave as you do?

Your behavior did not suddenly appear overnight but took a long time developing. You clearly have problems dealing with your emotions. Counseling will help you deal with the needs and emotions that you have lost touch with after years of numbing your mind with food and exercise to the point that you really have no idea anymore what it is you really hunger for. A trained counselor will be able to give you a better understanding of yourself, and if you find private counseling too costly, you should find out where your hospitals and community centers have group therapy.

Only when you have the courage to move away from food and weight preoccupation to find out who you really are is full recovery—physically and emotionally—possible. Until you stop obsessing about food and body image you will never feel in control, never feel nourished, and never feel fulfilled. One day you will learn to live life to the full again. When your period returns, or starts for the first time, it will not be seen as some kind of fearful omen, but a wonderful indication that your new life of health, self-discovery, and happiness has begun.

Treatment for Early Menopause and Amenorrhea that Is Irreversible

Sometimes, in very rare instances, primary or secondary amenorrhea is irreversible. This can be caused by congenital defects, such as the absence or abnormal function of the reproductive organs, or by disease, such as a tumor or an infection. In severe hypothalamic cases, such as chronic anorexia nervosa or bulimia, periods disappear forever because of the long-term distress the body has been placed in.

If you have early menopause, your period will not return either, but sometimes after menopause occurs, you may still have follicles and suddenly release an egg. This is an unlikely scenario, but fertility drugs may stimulate ovulation again. Early menopause is not always completely irreversible if follicles are still present or can be preserved, and you may still be able to conceive.

Patients in premature menopause or who are permanently amenorrheaic for other reasons will be prescribed replacement hormones or birth control pills. Estrogen is usually prescribed for bone strength and for cardiac and vaginal health. Sometimes higher levels of hormone replacement therapy will be prescribed because doctors believe that younger women are used to higher levels of estrogen. Others prescribe lower levels depending on your age. Hormonal therapy will protect against heart disease, osteoporosis, cancer, and other symptoms of female hormone deficiency. Therapy to help you come to terms with the situation will probably also be advised.

Summary

Amenorrhea can be caused by many pathological states, and medical evaluation usually leads to correct diagnosis. The role of your doctor should be to offer you reassurance that in time menses will return if proper lifestyle adjustments and/or hormonal therapy are used. Remember that in the great majority of cases amenorrhea does reverse itself either naturally or with treatment that is physical, psychological, or a mixture of both.

While you are being treated, and even after the condition has reversed itself, your doctor will probably want to keep a close check on you. Regular physical examinations, hormonal assessments, and checks on your diet and exercise levels may be necessary to prevent a reoccurrence and to guard against the major health risks of amenorrhea, osteoporosis, heart disease, and cancer.

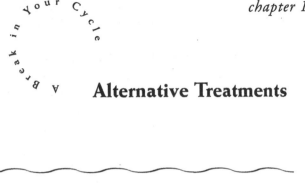

chapter 13

Alternative Treatments

THESE DAYS NATURAL OPTIONS FOR HEALTH AND WELL-being are extremely popular. In the last ten years or so, natural health care has enjoyed tremendous growth, and there are now many treatment options available to consumers. Also, the divide that used to exist between the natural and the orthodox approaches is no longer so wide, and learning and interaction are taking place between the two to offer the best health care treatment available.

Natural Versus Orthodox Medicine

Natural health care has always existed; it is as old as mankind. For centuries people have turned to the healing power of touch, to special diet, to herbal remedies, to hot and cold water to stimulate circulation, and to manipulating the body's energy fields to promote health and well-being.

Orthodox medicine does not have such a long history to prove its use. It did not begin to develop until the late nineteenth century. Often considered the medicine of the West, orthodox medicine stresses the importance of cure: finding a drug to kill a disease or to correct a chemical imbalance in the body. Doctors tend to be impersonal in their search for a quick answer to the problem and the belief that it can be fixed by medication. The problem, though, is that often in destroying what is harmful, drugs also destroy what is beneficial. Antibiotics are a case in point. They kill harmful bacteria that cause the infection, but at the same time they destroy the body's beneficial bacteria. Many drugs can also have unpleasant and dangerous side effects. Yet despite all this, there is much that is good about the orthodox approach. It has been and often is a life saver. It comes to its own in times of crisis, and millions of lives have been saved by it where natural medicine might have failed.

Should I See an Alternative Practitioner?

If you have a real understanding of your body, you will probably be able to understand whether you should go to a traditional or an orthodox doctor. Unfortunately, if you are amenorrheaic, it is likely that you have been making unhealthy lifestyle choices and are not really in tune with your body, so perhaps it would be advisable to see an orthodox doctor first to understand the clinical cause of the amenorrhea and to check that no underlying disease process is at work. After consulting with your doctor, then it may be time to investigate natural therapies to complement medication from your doctor.

Natural therapy could be very beneficial for those who need to reduce stress levels and make lifestyle and diet changes to prevent the problem continuing or recurring in the future. A natural healer, rather than an orthodox doctor, will be better qualified to look at your whole lifestyle, physical and emotional, determine where there is an imbalance, and show you how you can become actively involved in your own recovery.

Alternative Treatments Available

The sheer number of different therapies available can be quite overwhelming if you decide to seek help from alternative medicine. The following list mentions just some of the most popular treatments:

Acupressure	Homeopathic medicine
Acupuncture	Humor therapy
Alexander Technique	Hypnotherapy
Aromatherapy	Macrobiotics
Art therapy	Mediation
Ayurvedic medicine	Megavitamins
Chiropractic medicine	Mind-body control
Counseling	Music therapy
Dance therapy	Native American practices
Diet, nutrition, lifestyle changes	Naturopathic medicine
Guided imagery	Nutritional supplements
Herbal medicine	Oriental medicine

Osteopathy
Past life therapy
Prayer therapy
Psychotherapy
Reflexology
Relaxation techniques

Shamanism
Tai Chi
Therapeutic touch
Tibetan medicine
Yoga

Which one to choose? Which one works best? Unfortunately there is no answer to give. Different therapies work for different women, and it may be a process of trial and error for you until you find out what works best for you. It would be wise to read about the various options available so you understand the principles behind them before you go for a consultation. Some will appeal to you more than others. If you are going for a consultation, make sure you check out the experience, qualifications, and background of the practitioner you visit. There are a lot of charlatans out there trying to cash in on people's vulnerability and the current popularity of alternative therapy.

Many women suffering from amenorrhea have found a cure in alternative therapies. Again, it is probably wiser to try it alongside, or after, treatment by a conventional doctor. You first need to ensure that there is no underlying disease at work that needs immediate treatment and to determine if you need hormone-related therapy to counteract the side effects of amenorrhea. You also need to make absolutely sure that the natural therapy you choose to pursue is as safe as it sounds. The following sections outline some alternative options often used to treat amenorrhea and menstrual dysfunction.

Naturopathy

The term *naturopathy* originated in the late nineteenth century, but the practice can be traced back thousands of years. People have always believed that healing will occur naturally in the human body if it is given what it truly needs: clean water, a balanced diet, fresh air, sunlight, exercise, and adequate sleep. Rather than finding disease and killing it, the body is helped to establish its own state of good health with various recommendations and techniques. The emphasis is on prevention rather than cure and on strengthening the body to fight disease. The naturopath's code can therefore be summed up by one simple statement: the body is self-healing.

The body strives toward health and has power to heal itself. We can see this ourselves when a scar forms over a wound or body temperature adjusts naturally or our immune system fights disease itself. We are our own physicians. Problems only occur when the body is not treated with respect or the mind is in a state of crisis. In order to be self-healing, both body and mind must be healthy, balanced, and well nourished. That is why almost all forms of natural healing focus on proper nourishment through a balanced diet, cleansing toxins that have accumulated in the body, or in balancing the flow of energy through the body and reducing levels of stress in your life to gain emotional contentment.

A poor diet and unhealthy lifestyle often are what cause disease in the first place, so natural practitioners look at the person as a whole rather than just focusing on the problem. They recognize that you are not just a cold or a flu, but that your illness will affect all areas of your life—physical, mental, and spiritual. You will be shown how to restore your body to health so it can fight the disorder itself, and you will be educated about how to prevent recurrence of illness. Drugs, surgery, and harmful substances will never be used on the body.

When you visit a practitioner of natural medicine you will probably have a consultation. Here you will notice the difference from orthodox medicine. The consultation may take longer and the doctor will want to know about your whole lifestyle, not just your amenorrhea. Your emotional state as well as your physical state will be discussed so that what is negatively influencing your health can be determined. Both a naturopath and an orthodox doctor will regard your amenorrhea as a symptom. The orthodox doctor will directly attack what is causing the problem and try to correct it with medication. A naturopath recognizes that no drug can be given for malnutrition or unhealthy lifestyle and, more often than not, missing periods is your body's way of way of telling you that you need to make a change in lifestyle and diet. Recommendations about how you can restore your body and your reproductive cycle to good health will be made.

Usually the consultation and diagnosis will be free. The recommendations, which might include treatments such as dietary supplements or herbal remedies, are what you pay for. If you think that the treatment is too costly, it probably is, so shop around until you find something you can afford, or learn about alternative medicine methods yourself. There are many lively and informative books available on the market that can give you the knowledge you require. Do be very careful though. Just because natural medicine says it is natural does not always mean it is good for you. Many natural therapies that are available haven't been properly researched or properly labeled. Be wary of exaggerated miracle cures. Some treatments can cause negative reactions. Socrates was killed by hemlock, remember! To be safe, make sure you check thoroughly for safety before you take any herbs or dietary supplements or have physical therapy.

Ayurvedic Medicine

This is a practice for the cultivation and harnessing of internal energy for the enhancement of energy flow in the body. If you are amenorrheaic you will learn about energy points in your body and how being amenorrheaic creates a blockage to this natural flow. You will be taught various techniques to release the blocked energy and (hopefully) restore your periods.

Herbal Medicine

Herbal medicine is an integral part of Chinese medicine, as it is in many other cultures. Your herbalist will work to match the therapeutic characteristics and nature of herbs to formulate a prescription to meet your needs. Herbal medicine is quite similar to traditional Western medicine in that many prescription drugs originate from plants. After consultation, plant remedies or herbal teas to trigger the menstrual process, to help regulate hormones, and to nourish the body will be prescribed if you are amenorrheaic. Native American practices use squaw vine as the herb for amenorrhea.

Acupuncture, Tai Chi, and Yoga

Acupuncture is a method of correcting energy blocks in your body that cause menstrual dysfunction. Healing and functioning are promoted through inserting needles at precise points on the body. Meridians, channels of energy, run like currents throughout the body. When blockage in one part of a channel occurs, it impedes the flow of others. Acupuncture removes the blockage and revives the usual flow through the meridians, restoring balance.

Acupressure works along similar principles. Tai Chi and yoga also emphasize the importance of correct energy flow in the body and how ill health results where there is an imbalance or a blockage.

Aromatherapy

Aromatherapy is the therapeutic use of essential oils, which are highly concentrated substances distilled from aromatic herbs, flowers, and trees. They are chemically complex and contain hormonelike properties, vitamins and minerals, and natural antiseptics. Documented use of some of these dates back thousands of years; the ancient Egyptians and then the Greeks used them, and many of their uses have been scientifically tested. When breathed in, essential oils send a direct message to the brain, where they can affect the endocrine and hormonal systems via the hypothalamus, which is particularly relevant for amenorrheaics. The oils can also affect you through your skin if used in a massage, compress, or bath. Tiny molecules of oil pass through the skin and reach the blood and lymphatic system where they are carried to where they are needed.

Essential oils can have a beneficial effect on menstrual dysfunction. To get the oils that are right for you, obtain a custom-made blend from a professional aromatherapist or learn about the practice yourself.

Homeopathy

The homeopathic principle was invented in 1790 by Samuel Hahnemann. He saw in his medical practice that blood letting and the use of strong drugs weakened the body. Homeopaths advocate the use of very small doses of medicine. The idea is to stimulate the patient's immune system and defense capacity—the overall resistance. Finding the precise individual substance required is the art of homeopathy, but other factors such as stress management and exercise are included in treatment, which takes into account both body and mind.

More and more doctors are beginning to refer patients to homeopathic physicians. Homeopathic treatments can effectively treat menstrual problems and the various psychological problems commonly associated with menstruation.

Nutritional Therapy

Nutritional deficiencies will be seen by nutrition specialists as the cause of your amenorrhea. A balanced diet will be recommended, food to which there is an allergic reaction will be eliminated, and various vitamin and mineral supplements will be suggested. Typical recommendations might include eating food rich in zinc, such as fish; taking vitamin E supplements; adding vitamin B complex, which is found in wheat germ; getting enough protein, or including seaweed in your diet.

Physical Therapies

Various measures such as warm sitz baths or using clay compresses or caster oil packs on your lower abdomen will be recommended to stimulate the body's circulation and trigger menstrual function.

Stress Reduction and Mind-Body Control

Since amenorrhea is often stress-related, careful attention will be paid to eliminating stressful situations from your life (such as a busy schedule or an exercise or food addiction). To help you cope better with the stress, relaxation techniques such as meditation, paying attention to your breathing, and yoga may be recommended by specialists in this field, as will getting enough fresh air and keeping regular eating, sleeping, and bathing habits.

Psychotherapy

Emotional stress may disturb the hypothalamic-pituitary-ovarian axis and produce amenorrhea. Recognizing the strong mind-body link that exists, counseling or psychotherapy may be the best approach to help you come to terms with the anxiety, pain, and unresolved issues in your life that may be inhibiting menstrual function. Other therapies to deal with the underlying emotional issues at stake with something as complex as the menstrual cycle include mind-body work, visualization, art, music, or dance therapy, and guided visualization.

Summary

Alternative remedies tend to work on the principle that if you are amenorrheic your body is warning you that there is an imbalance in your life. Because you are treated as a whole person—mind, body, and spirit—you are more likely to come to a greater understanding of your body and yourself than if you were treated by orthodox medicine alone. You will learn that if mind and body are happy and nourished, your chance of being healthy and having normal menstrual function significantly increases. This realization should prompt you to look at your life and make some of the positive lifestyle changes recommended in the next chapter.

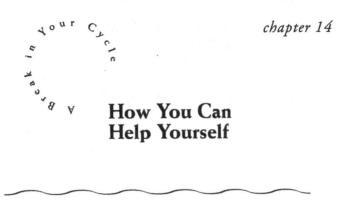

chapter 14

How You Can Help Yourself

AMENORRHEA IS NOT A DISEASE BUT A CONDITION. IT should be clear by now that this is no reason to neglect it. Month after month your absent periods are telling you that you are not healthy.

Step One: See a Doctor

You may be tempted to avoid seeing a doctor, hoping that your periods will come back as mysteriously as they disappeared. This is unwise. Your periods vanished for a reason, and you need to find out why. The importance of seeing a doctor, if you have been amenorrheaic for more than six months, cannot be underestimated. Why? The reasons have all been mentioned before, but they are so important I will stress them again.

1. Your body is in a state of crisis. Women were designed to have periods.
2. You need to make sure that what is causing your amenorrhea is not a dangerous disease or tumor.
3. You need to determine if you are in early menopause, and if you are, you will need medication to avoid many of the risks and unpleasant side effects of menopause.
4. You may be estrogen-deficient, which makes your risk of developing heart disease and osteoporosis very high.
5. You are in danger of developing cancer of the womb.

Step Two: Cultivate a Balanced, Healthy Lifestyle

In an ideal world we would all be the best judge of what is good for our health, but unfortunately in today's fast-moving society this is no longer the case. We eat badly, sleep too little, work too hard, don't get enough fresh air, and keep putting off that doctor's appointment. We have become so used to feeling unhealthy—suppressing and denying the messages our body sends us—that we don't really know what feeling good is anymore. Our bodies, however, have a way of showing us that our determination is wrong. We can only go on punishing ourselves for so long. Eventually the body will rebel with ill health and demand that you pay it more attention. Amenorrhea is your body crying out for help. It is asking you to take a look at your lifestyle. Are you going to listen?

Aside from seeking medical advice, cultivating a balanced, healthy lifestyle is how you can best help yourself. Our bodies need a proper diet, fresh air and exercise, rest and sleep, as well as regular medical checkups. If we paid more attention to these basics we would all feel better and complaints of ill health would not be so widespread.

Nutrition

The human body relies on food to build its tissues and provide the energy needed to maintain the living processes such as digestion, respiration, and circulation. We have already seen that if the food taken in is inadequate, or lacks the essential nutrients, the body cannot supply enough energy to maintain the menstrual cycle.

Fast food, junk food, and other foods with the nutrients processed, frozen, and squeezed out of them are the staples of our society. Our bodies need certain essential nutrients: proteins, carbohydrates, fats, vitamins, minerals, water, and other trace elements. The quality and balance of these nutrients is very important. Eating more or less than is necessary will result in weight fluctuations. An insufficient supply of the nutrients the body needs is dangerous both in the long and short term. Good health—and good menstrual health—depends on a good diet, and that means a diet that is balanced.

A balanced diet is one that contains the right quality and the right quantity of food for you. How much you need will depend on your

FIGURE 2
Height/Weight Chart

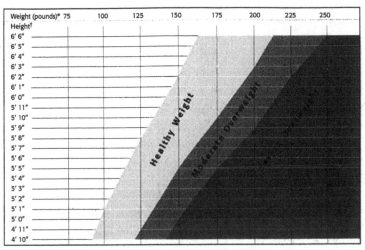

Source: *Report of the Dietary Guidelines Advisory Committee on the Dietary Guidelines for Americans,* 1995.
* without clothes; † without shoes

build and how active you are. Height and weight charts (see Figure 2) only give you a vague idea of your ideal weight for your height. These charts are typically based on mortality data from people who buy life insurance, not from disease and mortality statistics from the general population. You should focus on your health, exercise levels, and your diet rather than on your body weight

If you want to get some idea of how healthy your weight is for your height, the Body Mass Index (BMI) is a more sophisticated height-weight correlation than the charts. To figure out your BMI, multiply your weight in pounds by 700. Then divide this number by the square of your height in inches. For example, if you are 64 inches tall and weigh 140 pounds, multiply 140 x 700 and get 98,000. Then divide 98,000 by the square of 64, which is 4,096, to get your BMI: 23.9. For men and women a healthy BMI is between 20 and 25. If you are way above 25 or way below 20, then a balanced diet, combined with weight loss or weight gain, will be an essential part of your recovery.

Knowing what foods contain which nutrients and why they are needed will help you plan a balanced diet.

CARBOHYDRATES Carbohydrates, our main source of energy, are found in starch, in sugar, and in fiber. Starch is a good source of carbohydrates and is found in bread, potatoes, rice, pasta, and cereal. Carbohydrates are used by the body as a source of energy and can be stored as glycogen for later use. Excess carbohydrate is converted to fat. Sugars are not a good source of carbohydrate if they are found in sucrose (table sugar), but natural sugars, found in fruits and vegetables, are. Fiber provides little energy but is very important because it plays an important part in regular bowel movements. Good sources are whole-meal bread and pasta, vegetables, and fruit. Food that contains starch and fiber should account for about 60 percent of your diet.

PROTEINS Proteins are the substances that build tissues for growth and repair. They are also an aid in reducing menstrual problems. They are found in foods like lean meat, poultry, fish, eggs, milk and milk products, beans, nuts, yeast, grains, and wheat germ. Protein should account for about 10 percent of a healthy diet.

FATS Fats keep the body functions working and should account for about 30 percent of our diet. Saturated fats are mainly of animal origin and are found in meat, milk, butter, and cheese. They should be taken in moderation since they can raise blood cholesterol to dangerous levels. Polyunsaturated fats tend to occur in plants and soybean oil and they tend to lower blood cholesterol.

WATER Our bodies are about two-thirds water, so the intake and distribution of fluid is important for our well-being. If the body is deprived of water, blood volume is reduced and does not circulate to the tissues as effectively. The brain is most affected, and you might feel dizzy. You will almost certainly feel fatigued if you are dehydrated. The solution is to drink enough water. Six to eight glasses a day is recommended.

MINERALS Calcium is needed for bone growth, healthy teeth, blood clotting, and iron absorption, and it is an aid for relieving menstrual problems. It is found in milk, milk products, egg yolks, green vegetables, and shellfish.

Iodine is an aid in regulating energy use in the body. It is found in seafood and seaweed.

Iron is the basic component of blood hemoglobin and prevents anemia. It is found in meat, green vegetables, yeast, and wheat germ.

Magnesium is involved in the normal functioning of the brain, spinal cord, and nerves and is an aid in bone formation and reducing menstrual problems. It is found in milk, grains, vegetables, fruits, and cereals.

Phosphorus is required for bone growth, strong teeth, and energy transformation. It is found in milk, yogurt, yeast, and wheat germ.

Potassium is needed for healthy nerves and muscles. It is found in milk, fruit, and vegetables.

Sodium is the main chemical that maintains adequate water and cells in the body. It is found in table salt, milk, meat, and most canned goods.

Zinc plays an essential role in the development of reproductive organs and in the body's enzyme systems. It is found in egg yolks, milk, nuts, peas, and beans.

VITAMINS Vitamin A fights infection and prevents dry skin and poor bone growth. It is found in vegetables, milk, butter, margarine, and egg yolks.

Vitamin B complex (B_1) is essential for the nervous system and is found in wheat, bran, yeast, and beans.

Vitamin B_2 is needed for growth. It is found in milk, meat, eggs, and leafy vegetables.

Niacin is an aid in preventing disease and for a glowing complexion. You can find it in milk, eggs, cheeses, and fish.

Vitamin B_{12}, for healthy skin and a healthy nervous system, is in milk, eggs, cheese, and fish.

Folic acid is for cell production and healthy skin. It is found in leafy green vegetables, chicken, liver, and kidneys.

Vitamin C, found in green vegetables and citrus fruits, prevents colds, heals wounds, and is essential for normal metabolism and the reduction of menstrual problems.

Vitamin D, for bone growth and calcium absorption, is also an aid for reducing menstrual difficulties. It is found in tuna fish, eggs, butter, and cheese.

Vitamin E promotes blood clotting and is found in milk, vegetables, liver, rice, and bran.

Vitamin K is active in maintaining the involuntary nervous system, the vascular system, and involuntary muscles. It is found in wheat germ, vegetable oil, whole-grain breads, and cereals.

CAFFEINE AND ALCOHOL Reducing or eliminating the amount of caffeine and alcohol is also vital if a balanced diet is your goal. Alcohol can cause high blood pressure and caffeine can cause stress, fatigue, headaches, and lack of energy. Caffeine and alcohol also deplete the body of water and minerals because they have a diuretic effect.

Anyone who regularly misses out on their nutrients is putting their health at risk because the body lacks the vital elements it requires to function normally. A normal menstrual cycle has specific dietary needs, and if there is dysfunction it may well be due to some kind of nutrient deficiency. Women who are amenorrheaic should ensure that they get all the nutrients required in their food or—second best—via supplements from drug and health stores. Healthy amounts of protein and vitamins B, C, D, and E should be a priority as should getting enough iron, zinc, calcium, and magnesium and avoiding foods rich in sodium, which can cause bloating and fatigue.

Although vitamin and mineral supplements can never take the place of a balanced diet, they can sometimes be beneficial. Estrogen-deficient women do report finding relief from taking Vitamin E or evening primrose oil. Herbs can also be helpful. Plants like soybeans, lima beans, chick-peas, flaxseed, and linseed are whole grains rich in plant estrogen.

The timing of meals is also very significant. Sometimes eating three meals a day will not suit you and you will feel better having several light snacks to avoid hypoglycemia, which occurs when the body goes from the fed state to the fasting state and you feel unwell. When food is spread out over the day with light, regular snacking, there is a better utilization of calories and you feel better because you have a constant supply of energy.

Malnutrition, in combination with an inappropriate body weight for your height and age, will almost certainly negatively influence normal menstrual function. We really are what we eat. If your diet is poor and lacks sufficient nutrients, your health—mentally, emotionally, and physically—will be poor too.

Sleep and Relaxation

Lack of sleep or too much sleep will make you feel fatigued and depressed. If your energy is low you may be sleep-deprived. Sleep is biologically necessary. Most of us need around eight hours a night. If we do not get it, we will not function well and it will affect our mood. Too much sleep can also get you out of condition, so you need to discover what is best for you. Sleep is vital for optimum brain power, and without it we quickly become depressed, irritated, stressed, and fuzzy-headed.

Relaxation is almost as important as sleep. Many women lead frantic, busy lives and when they do finally get the time to relax they don't know how. We work hard, eat fast, play competitively, and toss and turn in our sleep. Our calendars are full and we get tense if we don't achieve all that we said we would in one day at work and at home. Living in a constant state of stress like this will eventually have a negative effect on menstrual function.

If a healthy, balanced lifestyle is ever to be cultivated, relaxation—taking time out—is essential. Relaxation is time for you. Each of us must find different ways to relax. Walking in the fresh air, watching a movie, reading a good book, seeing friends, drawing a picture, and playing an instrument are all ways to relax. Relaxation time gives you the opportunity to recharge the batteries and focus on what makes you feel good. Unfortunately, many women tend to neglect time and space for themselves. Many find it impossible to relax at all, and they are the ones most prone to menstrual dysfunction because of high stress levels in their lives.

If you have problems relaxing, you need to learn how to take time out. One way to do this is to relax your whole body slowly, muscle by muscle. There are many tapes on the market that can help you through this process. Slowing down your breathing also gives you a chance to calm down. Techniques like meditation and yoga can also have astonishing results on women who are stressed and tense. Try this simple routine: Choose a focus word or phrase, such as *peace* or *happy.* Sit quietly, and relax your body by tensing and releasing your muscles and breathing deeply. Say the focus word each time you exhale. If you lose your concentration, simply return your thoughts to the word. Try this for just five minutes at first and then gradually increase the time. Do the routine at least once a day. Such relaxation exercises done regularly can slow your breathing rate, calm your brain wave rhythms, and lower your blood pressure. Yoga also can relax tense muscles, teach you better breathing, lower your blood pressure, decrease your heart rate, and divert your mind from stress.

When you feel stressed you could also try counting to ten before you react or repeat to yourself some positive affirmations like "I am in control." Soothing music can also be beneficial. So can soaking in a hot tub, laughing more, interacting with others, and cultivating outside interests and diversions from the routine. There are so many delightful ways to relax. You should not think of it as time lost; it is time gained. When you return to your routine you will feel refreshed, energized, and in control, and you will have a better perspective on things.

If you are amenorrheaic and lead a highly stressful life, make time for more relaxation. Stress and lack of sleep not only affect menstrual function but your whole body. There is nothing heroic about pushing yourself to the limits mentally, emotionally, and physically. You will feel drained, irritable, and fatigued. Instead of achieving more you will achieve less. Instead of feeling good you will feel unhealthy. Instead of having periods you will become amenorrheaic.

Exercise

One of the most effective ways to relax is exercise, as long as it is not taken to the extremes. Too much exercise can have a disastrous effect on menstrual function. If you are exercising to excess and are amenorrheaic as well, now is the time to gradually cut down and get some sense of perspective on your life. Professional and amateur athletes should talk to doctors and coaches so that the problem is dealt with right away, before health completely fails.

A moderate amount of exercise is beneficial and can ease stress. Exercise is essential to a healthy life, and regular exercise for fitness has many benefits. It can help us keep our heart and lungs in good condition, improve circulation, promote energy and health, remove toxic substances from the body, improve posture, and improve our self-image, and it helps reduce stress, anxiety, and depression. Vigorous aerobic exercise can reduce the level of pulse-quickening hormones released during stress and stimulate a feeling of well-being. Even a thirty-minute walk around the block can reduce anxiety. Try to schedule the exercise of your choice—running, swimming, walking—several times a week for thirty minutes.

Relationships

With the disintegration of the community and family unit, loneliness, isolation, and lack of intimacy is widespread. Partnerships with both sexes, both sexual and nonsexual, are important for good health. Our lives find meaning not only through how we feel about ourselves but in our relationships with others. No woman is an island. To be happy, we need others, and to feel fulfilled, we need many kinds of different relationships.

One of the best ways you can help yourself is to try, even though it may not come easily to you, to build successful relationships with others. These relationships, however, should not be ones that drain you but ones that make you feel good about yourself. If your friends are only interested in themselves or take you for granted, then they are not friends. If you believe that friendship is all about your own needs being fulfilled, then you are not a friend. Friendship is about giving and receiving, and it is based on the capacity to accept as well as to give love and respect.

Regular Medical Checkups

Doctors advise women to have an internal (pelvic or gynecological) examination at least once a year, starting in their late teens, and twice a year if they are over forty. If you do this your doctor will be able to diagnose and treat amenorrhea before it becomes a long-term condition and puts your health at risk. Going regularly to your doctor will also give you reassurance that your reproductive organs are not diseased and are functioning normally, and that hormone levels are stable.

Step Three: Listen to Your Body

Emotional and psychological stress does affect our bodies physically. We can become ill because of distress. But the opposite of this is true as well. The creation of health and well-being is both physical, emotional, and mental. How we think and feel will play an active part in our recovery.

Our thoughts, our feelings, and our brains communicate with the rest of our body, influencing the nervous and endocrine system, our immune system, and the organs of our body. You could say that the mind is not just in the brain but is located throughout the body. We are what we think. Everything we think, everything we feel, will resonate through our entire body. If there is a problem with one of our organs, our "body mind" is speaking to us through it. We should pay attention to our body when it speaks and learn to listen more to the warnings it sends us.

Many women who are amenorrheaic have somewhere along the line lost touch with their body's needs, stopped paying attention to how their body feels, and ignored the signals that have been sent. Too many times the need to eat, the need to rest, the need to relax, the need to cry has been suppressed or denied. The body now resorts to more drastic measures to try to send a message, and periods will stop.

Learning to listen to your body may take some getting used to, but in time you will begin to sense when it is sending you messages. Try to listen. If it hurts, stop. If you are tired, rest. If you are hungry or thirsty, eat and drink. If you are full, stop eating. If you feel happy, smile. If you feel sad, cry.

Step Four: Reconnect with Your Emotions

Many of us find it hard to understand or feel our emotions properly. Emotions are important because they help us experience life more fully. It is not always easy to trust our emotions; sometimes they seem very illogical, and we have been conditioned to delay or deny their expression. Yet the very nature of emotions is to be illogical. Sometimes, for instance, our body just feels the need to cry or to be angry. Instead of questioning and denying our emotions, we should simply allow ourselves to feel what our bodies want us to feel.

We may be frightened of so-called negative emotions such as anger, fear, and sadness, but the expression of all our emotions will lead to improved physical and mental health. This is not to say that you need to act on them all the time. We simply can't go around doing exactly what we feel, but we should acknowledge that these emotions exist because when negative emotions are not expressed they cause even greater stress. When they are bottled up they affect our whole bodies, especially the immune system, because we are not allowing ourselves to feel or act as we should. Our emotions are messages that come from our inner wisdom. If they are not worked through, the biochemical effect that suppressed emotions have on our immune system will cause physical problems.

A Break in Your Cycle

Feeling and expressing our emotions is the only real way we have to acknowledge that our life matters to us. They show us how important our life is to us, and how important it should be to those around us. Sometimes these emotions will cause us pain and distress, but negative emotions also signal the need for some kind of change in our lives. They require us to act, to change the situation that is causing distress, to rebel against what we see as an injustice, to move on with our lives. Negative emotions are not bad emotions; they can be necessary for us to grow and develop.

The only really bad emotion is an emotion that gets stuck or is unacknowledged. Many amenorrheaics have problems dealing with their emotions and understanding themselves. The tendency is to bottle up negative emotions and withdraw from the challenge of personal development. The need for change is denied, and so the body mirrors this stalemate by standing still and stopping menses.

One of the ways you can help yourself if you are amenorrheaic is to try to deal with your emotions. You may be so used to repression and denial that you find this impossible to do alone, so you will need the help of a therapist, but somehow you must learn that life involves change and growth.

Amenorrhea draws attention to the organs that make you who you are. It is an expression of your crisis of development. The problem is usually not just physical, but is related to how you feel about yourself as a woman. The wisdom in your body is telling you that this is the area of your life that most needs attention and where there is some kind of emotional problem. Frightened or repelled by what you think being a woman means, you don't really know who or what you are. Focusing on why you feel the way you do about being a woman will take great courage. If you have been shutting out challenge and growth, at times it may seem like facing a black hole, but self-awareness will only come when you allow yourself to experience fully all your emotions, both negative and positive.

The belief system that you have about being a woman may have set the stage for your amenorrhea. The only way to improve your health is to change the way you think about yourself. Individual self-development—finding out who you are—will be a quest that will take up the rest of your life, but only by engaging in that quest is the possibility of fulfillment and happiness within your reach. It will never be within your reach if you deny negative emotions, deny change and growth, deny self-expression, deny the significance of menstruation, and deny becoming the beautiful and unique woman you were meant to be.

Summary

A doctor may help you get your periods back, but ultimately the health of your reproductive system, your body, your mind, and your emotions lies in your hands. Your amenorrhea need not be forever and ever. You and no one else are in control of your life. You do not have to feel stressed, do not have to be malnourished, and do not have to feel anxious unless you choose to. And you do not, unless you are in menopause or have some serious disorder, have to miss periods either.

A Break in Your Cycle

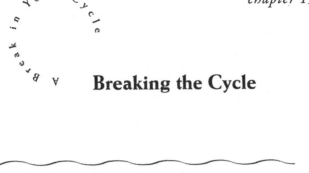

chapter 15

Breaking the Cycle

TO FULFILL OUR BIOLOGICAL ROLE AS CHILD BEARERS,
we are given reproductive organs. When we reach puberty, a lining
will be prepared within our wombs. If no pregnancy occurs, the lining is broken down and removed from our bodies in menstruation.
We can expect this to happen every month for about thirty years of
our life until we reach menopause. This is the normal female reproductive cycle. Amenorrheaic women break that cycle.

Considering that menstruation is a subject of universal importance, ensuring the continuation of the human race, it is incredible
that in our open-minded society attitudes about the female cycle remain Victorian. It is still a subject that causes embarrassment.
Finding the word *menstruation* hard to say, we have a whole vocab-
ulary of words that refer to it in other ambiguous ways. Some are
factual and uninteresting like *period* or *coming on;* more descriptive,
like *the blues* or *the time of the month;* some are familiar like *Charlie*
or *Archie;* some are ridiculous like *the reds are coming;* and some are
an expression of disgust, like the much used *the curse.* It is no sur-
prise then, in a society that is still so little prepared to understand or
value the normal menstrual cycle, that menstrual dysfunction and
how it can impact a woman's life are undervalued.

Of all the menstrual problems, one of the most neglected is
amenorrhea. Few of us are even familiar with the term. We are partly
to blame for this neglect. Too often we bear suffering without seeking help and advice. Unsympathetic doctors, who dismiss women's
problems as "all in the mind" or as not really something to be concerned about, have not helped. You might have been told that unless you wanted children there was nothing to worry about, or that

it is quite normal to miss periods if you are an athlete.

It took centuries for measures to be taken to relieve the pains of childbirth, and even longer for synthetic hormones to be developed to help with period problems. Thankfully, widespread recognition and treatment of conditions like amenorrhea should not take as long. There are encouraging signs of a developing medical understanding of amenorrhea. Gradually it is being acknowledged that amenorrhea carries with it serious health risks that should not be ignored. Better treatment options and advice are more readily available than ever before.

Progress is certainly being made medically, but the emotional impact of menstrual dysfunction is still neglected by doctors. Missing periods is far more than a physical condition. Periods, sexuality, and identity are all linked in a woman's mind. How she feels about her menstrual cycle reveals how she feels about herself as a woman.

Not having periods has great emotional significance, the importance of which should not be underestimated, regardless of what is causing the amenorrhea. It is normal to have periods, and you may be terrified that something is seriously wrong with you when you don't. Emotionally, you exhaust yourself. Have you got a tumor? Has menopause come early? Are you pregnant? Are you infertile? You need reassurance from your doctor. Being told to come back in a few months to see if the condition reverses itself, or being given a pack of pills will not give you peace of mind.

If amenorrhea is irreversible, or if there is early menopause, how are you to cope emotionally? Hormonal therapy will not make you look any older, but you might still feel scared and uncertain about how you should regard yourself in a world where traditional ideas about a woman's role as fertile child bearer are deeply ingrained. You have to face the difficult task of redefining yourself as a woman. This transition is something all of us face when we reach menopause, but you will be going through all this without the support of your age group, and without the knowledge and experience an older woman has gained. Even if you never intended to have children, there will still be a sense of loss, and you will need time to grieve for that loss and rebuild your life anew. Counseling, advice, and help should be more readily available.

Or you may be suffering from some of the unpleasant side effects of conditions like polycystic ovary syndrome and elevated prolactin levels. Facial hair and acne or leaking breasts embarrass you and make you feel unattractive. And there is always the hidden fear of infertility and cancer. Apart from treatment, what you need—but don't always get—is understanding and empathy.

Then there are those of us who have unconsciously played an active part in creating the amenorrheaic state. We eat poorly, exercise too much, and are constantly stressed out. We may fear or resent being female. Perhaps we feel inferior in some way and think that without the burden of menstruation we can be more like men. Or perhaps the female form terrifies us. Our loathing of female fat may be so deeply ingrained that we are prepared to risk our health to avoid it. Or maybe we want our lives to stand still. We may want to be like Sleeping Beauty and never really face the challenges of adult life. Do we feel ashamed and revolted by menstruation? Or is the obsessive need to work hard for a job, or train for a sport, so overwhelming that we lose all sense of perspective about our lives?

If your amenorrhea is stress-induced, missed periods express your crisis of identity and your emotional confusion. Something has gone very wrong in the formation of your belief system. In a world that expects so much from women in all spheres of their lives, being a woman is something that causes conflict within you, and the drama of conflict and confusion is played out in your body, the only place where you feel you have any control. You push your body to impossible limits, and periods stop. You need help understanding that only by facing challenge and change and making mistakes will you be able to learn, grow, and find a sense of identity. As long as you remain amenorrheaic, you will never learn who and what you are. You will stand still.

With something as complex as amenorrhea, there will always be underlying emotional issues involved. Treating the physical problem alone is not enough. Whatever the unconscious motivation, recovery from amenorrhea will never be complete until the emotional issues, often neglected by doctors, are addressed too. Too many times the problem is diagnosed and treatment is started without an appreciation of the underlying emotional issues at stake. Getting your periods back will not change how you feel. Emotional and spiritual healing must also take place if recovery is to be complete.

There are very encouraging signs that conventional medicine is beginning to take into account the importance of how we think and how we feel, recognizing it as a major part of the recovery process, but there is still some way to go. You may be lucky enough to get reassurance, advice, and counseling, but more often than not you must become your own inner physician. If you have menstrual dysfunction, your "body mind" is calling your attention to the menstrual cycle for a reason. If you do not listen to what your body is saying, your health—mental, emotional, and physical—will suffer. Your body is telling you that it is time to acknowledge the importance of your emotions, to come to terms with your sexuality, to look at how you relate to other people, to review the way you think about yourself as a woman.

A very positive development in modern medical science is that the emphasis is finally shifting toward an appreciation of the differences between the male and female body, and the vital role hormones play in our physical and emotional lives. It can only be hoped that this move away from the male-centered approach will encourage us to see how, in our quest for equality with men, we have undervalued our unique differences from men. Mistakenly thinking that being equal is to be like men, we have not celebrated our female form, but regulated and organized it through the pill, diet, exercise, denial, and amenorrhea. We have overemphasized discipline at the expense of our creativity and spontaneity. It is time to break that cycle. The only way for us to be truly equal is to stop trying to be the same as men. We will only find true equality when we start to value, respect, and give expression to what is unique about ourselves as women.

The increase of menstrual dysfunction as we move into the twenty-first century shows how many of us are in danger of losing touch with our uniqueness. It is time now to stop controlling, punishing, dismissing, or ignoring our bodies and to reconnect once more with our femininity and our bodily rhythms and acknowledge the powerful role feelings play in our lives. Surely now in this age, with all the wonderful opportunities available to us, we should understand that being a woman is not limited to the definition of daughter, wife, mother, or grandmother, but about feeling creative and fulfilled in our own lives and contributing to society in the ways in which each one of us is uniquely suited.

bibliography/
suggested reading

Aron, David. 1995. "Pituitary Tumors: Current Concepts in Diagnosis and Management." *Western Journal of Scientific Medicine* 162 (4): 340.

Baird, David. 1997. "Amenorrhea." Review article. *The Lancet,* July 26, 350 (9073): 275.

Benyo, Richard. 1990. *The Exercise Fix: How the Aerobic Athlete's Compulsive Need for the Next Workout is Self-destructive.* Champaign, IL: Leisure Press.

Bonnick, Sydney Lou. 1997. *The Osteoporosis Handbook: Every Woman's Guide to Prevention and Treatment.* Dallas, TX: Taylor Publishing.

Borysenko, Joan. 1987. *Minding the Body, Mending the Mind.* New York: Bantam Books.

Borysenko, Joan. 1996. *A Woman's Book of Life: The Biology, Psychology and Spirituality of the Feminine Life Cycle.* New York: Riverhead Books.

Bruch, Hilde. 1978. *The Golden Cage: The Enigma of Anorexia Nervosa.* Cambridge, MA: Harvard University Press.

Chernin, Kim. 1981. *The Obsession: Reflections on the Tyranny of Slenderness.* New York: Harper and Row.

Chernin, Kim. 1994. *The Hungry Self: Women, Eating and Identity.* New York: HarperPerennial.

Chihal, Jane, and S. London, eds. "Menstrual Cycle Disorders." *Obstetrics and Gynecology Clinics of North America Journal* 17 (2).

Cohen, Sharon. 1994. "When Your Period Stops, Your Poor Eating Habits, Not Low Body Fat May Be the Culprit." *Shape* (Jan.): 40.

Collinge, William. 1987. *The American Holistic Health Association Complete Guide to Alternative Medicine.* New York: Warner Books.

Dietrich, Edward, and Carol Cohan. 1992. *Women and Heart Disease: What You Can Do to Stop the Number One Killer of American Women.* New York: Times Books.

Dreher, H. 1996. *Healing Mind, Healthy Woman.* New York: Henry Holt.

Epp, Susan. 1997. "The Diagnosis and Treatment of Athletic Amenorrhea." *Physician Assistant Journal* 21 (3): 129.

Forsyth, S. 1993. "Amenorrhea: What Your Body Is Trying to Tell You." *Cosmopolitan* (Oct.): 112, 114.

Franklin, Robert, and D. Brockman. 1990. *In Pursuit of Fertility: A Fertility Expert Tells You How to Get Pregnant.* New York: Henry Holt.

Frisch, R. E., and J. W. McArthur. 1975. "Menstrual Cycles: Fatness as a Determinant of Minimum Weight for Height Necessary for Their Maintenance and Onset." *Science* (185): 949–951.

Golden, Neville. 1994. "Amenorrhea in Anorexia Nervosa: Neuroendocrine Control of Hypothalamic Amenorrhea." *International Journal of Eating Disorders* 16 (1): 53.

Gravelle, Karen. 1996. *The Period Book: Everything You Don't Want to Know but Need to Ask.* New York: Walker and Co.

Hamilton, Linda. 1996. "How's Your Physical Timing?" *Dancer Magazine* (Nov.): 49.

Hatcher, Robert. 1994. *Contraceptive Technology.* New York: Irving Publishers.

Hetland, M. L., J. Haarbo, C. Christiansen, and T. Larsen. 1995. "Running Induces Menstrual Disturbances but Bone Mass is Unaffected in Amenorrheaic Women." *American Journal of Medicine* 7 (1): 53–60.

"HIV Linked to Menstrual Dysfunction." 1996. *AIDS Weekly Plus* (Sept. 9): 11.

Hoffman, Eileen. 1995. "Your Period: How Normal Is It?" *Cosmopolitan* (Mar.): 250.

Hogg, Anne Cahill. 1997. "Breaking the Cycle: Often Confused and Frustrated Sufferers of Amenorrhea Now Have Better Treatment Options." *American Fitness* (Jul./Aug.): 30.

Jacobowitz, Ruth. 1993. *150 Most Asked Questions About Osteoporosis: What Women Really Want to Know.* New York: Hearst Books.

Jansen, Robert. 1997. *Overcoming Infertility: A Compassionate Resource Guide for Getting Pregnant.* New York: WH Freeman.

Joy, Elisabeth. 1997. "What to Look For, What to Ask (Team Management of the Female Athletic Triad—Amenorrhea, Osteoporosis, Eating Disorders)." *Physician and Sports Medicine Journal* 25 (3): 94.

Kelting, E. G. 1988. "Exercise and Amenorrhea." *Cosmopolitan* (June): 170–172.

Kolodny, Nancy. 1992. *When Food's a Foe: How You Can Confront and Conquer Your Eating Disorders.* Boston, MA: Little, Brown and Company.

Lawrence, Marilyn, ed. 1987. *Fed Up and Hungry: Women, Oppression and Food.* New York: Bedrict.

Lee Vliet, Elizabeth. 1995. *Screaming to Be Heard: Hormonal Connections Women Suspect and Doctors Ignore.* New York: M Evans and Company.

Legato, M. J., and C. Coleman. 1991. *The Female Heart.* New York: Avon.

Levine, Hallie. 1997. "Am I Normal or Is Something Seriously Wrong?" *Cosmopolitan* (Aug.): 216.

McGarth, Ellen. 1992. *When Feeling Bad Is Good.* New York: Henry Holt and Company.

McGee, Carolyn. 1997. "Secondary Amenorrhea Leading to Osteoporosis: Incidence and Prevention." *The Nurse Practitioner Journal* 22 (5): 38.

Maddux, Hilary C. 1975. *Menstruation*. New Canann, CT: The Women's Library, Tobey Publishing Inc.

Matthews, Heidi. 1997. "Athletic Amenorrhea." *North Central College First Aider* 67 (2).

Michaud, Ellen, and Elizabeth Torg. 1995. *Total Health for Women: Prevent and Cure the 100 Health Care Problems Women Worry About Most*. Emmaus, PA: Rodale Press.

Murray, Michael. 1995. *Stress, Anxiety and Insomnia: How You Can Benefit from Diet, Vitamins, Minerals, Herbs and Exercise*. Rocklin, CA: Prima Publishing.

Nachtigall, Lila, and Joan Heilman. 1986. *Estrogen: The Facts Can Change Your Life*. New York: Harper and Row.

Northrup, Christine. 1995. *Women's Bodies, Women's Wisdom: Creating Physical and Emotional Healing*. New York: Bantam.

Notelovitz, Morris, and Marsha Ware. 1982. *Stand Tall: The Informed Women's Guide to Preventing Osteoporosis*. Gainesville, FL: Triad.

Orbach, Susie. 1986. *Hunger Strike: The Anorectic's Struggle as a Metaphor for Our Age*. New York: WW Norton.

Otis, C. L., and R. Goldingay. 1992. "A Crucial Period." *Shape* (Mar.): 50, 53.

"Premature Natural Menopause Can Be Devastating." 1995. *Menopause News* 5 (4): 1.

Redmond, Geoffrey P. 1995. *Androgenic Disorders*. New York: Raven Press.

Redmond, Geoffrey. 1995. *The Good News about Women's Hormones: Complete Information and Proven Solutions for the Most Common Hormonal Problems*. New York: Warner Books.

Roth, Geneen. 1982. *Feeding the Hungry Heart: The Experience of Compulsive Eating*. New York: NAL Books.

"Running Away from Motherhood." 1993. *Runners World* (Dec.): 18.

Scrambler, Annette. 1993. *Menstrual Disorders: The Experience of Illness.* London: Tavistock.

Sheehy, G. 1993. *Menopause: The Silent Passage.* New York: Pocket Books.

Shuttle, P., and P. Redgrove. 1990. *The Wise Wound: Myths, Realities and Meanings of Menstruation.* New York: Bantam.

Skolnick, Andrew A. 1996. "Health Pros Want New Rules for Girl Athletes." *Journal of the American Health Association* 275 (1): 22.

Smith, Angela. 1996. "The Female Athletic Triad: Causes, Diagnosis and Treatment (Disordered Eating, Amenorrhea and Osteoporosis)." *The Physician and Sports Medicine Journal* 24 (7): 67.

Speroff, Leon, R. Glass, and N. Kase. 1994. *Clinical Gynecologic Endocrinology and Infertility.* 5th ed. Baltimore: Williams and Wilkins.

"Starvation Diets Can Produce Health Risks." 1994. *Better Nutrition for Today's Living Journal* 56 (4): 22.

Van der Rol, R., and R. Verhoeven with an introduction by Anna Quindlen. 1995. *Anne Frank: Beyond the Diary.* New York: Puffin.

Vincent L. M. 1979. *Competing with the Sylph: Dancers and the Pursuit of the Ideal Body Form.* New York: Andrews and McMeel.

Weil, Andrew. 1995. *Understanding Conventional and Alternative Medicine.* Rev. ed. Boston: Houghton Mifflin.

index

heart disease
estrogen deficiency and
increase risk for, 95–96
herbal medicine, 137
hermaphrodite, 32
heroin, 68
hirsutism, 83–84
HIV, 47
Holy Anorexia (Bell), 71
homeopathy, 138
hormonal therapy, 129
hormones
effect on mood, 110–111
in follicular phase, 16
imbalance of, during amenorrhea, 92
importance of, 92
in luteal phase, 17
ovulation and, 16
Hunger Point (Medoff), 71
hymen
imperforate, 33–34
hyperprolactinemia, 124
hyperprolactinemic amenorrhea, 81–82
hypothalamic amenorrhea, 37,
83
hormonal therapy and, 129
stress and, 37, 128
hypothalamic-pituitary-
ovarian axis, 15
description of, 35–37
stress and, 39
hypothalamus
athletic training and, 57–58
function of, 35–37
gonadotrophin releasing
hormone, 16
hypothalamic amenorrhea,
83
in hypothalamic-pituitary-

ovarian axis, 35–37
problems with, 83
stress and, 39
hypothalamus gland
follicular phase, 16

I
imperforate hymen, 33–34
Indian medicine
view of amenorrhea and,
100
infertility
amenorrhea and, 100–101
early menopause and,
117–118
iron, 145
irreversible amenorrhea
adjusting to, 34–35
emotional effect of,
117–118
treatment for, 131–132

J
jobs
job insecurity, 44
overwork, 43–44
stressful professions, 43

K
kidney failure, 47

L
lesbianism, 112
Life Size (Shute), 71
lifestyle
cultivate balanced, healthy,
142–149
liver failure, 47
lower brain adhesions, 33
luteal phase, 17
emotions and, 17

9 781620 456972